I AM MORE
THAN MY INFERTILITY

htt
Printe
First pri
Lombardo,
I Am More Tha
Personal Breakt
ISBN: 978-0-980026

First in a series – I Am More

http://www.IAmMore.net

http://www.marinalombardo.com

p://www.lindaparkerbooks.com

d in the United States of America

ting 2007

Marina and Parker, Linda J.

n My Infertility 7 Proven Tools for Turning a Life Crisis into a
hrough / by Marina Lombardo and Linda J. Parker.

6-0-3

I AM MORE

THAN MY INFERTILITY

7 Proven Tools for Turning a Life Crisis into a Personal Breakthrough

Part of the Marina Lombardo series:

I Am More©

Seeds of Growth Press
Orlando, Florida

Like the crocus, it will burst into bloom;
it will rejoice greatly and shout for joy. Isaiah 35:2 (NIV)

With our deepest appreciation...

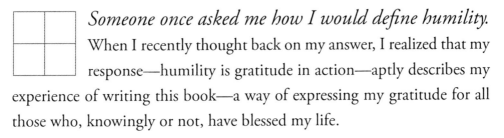

Someone once asked me how I would define humility. When I recently thought back on my answer, I realized that my response—humility is gratitude in action—aptly describes my experience of writing this book—a way of expressing my gratitude for all those who, knowingly or not, have blessed my life.

First and foremost, my husband, who has always been my biggest cheerleader, and encouraged me to keep writing from the days when I would read to him from my journal entries. My family, and especially my kids, who have been my personal tour guides on the adventure of motherhood. To *Conceive Magazine's* Kim Hahn, who invited me to take my message out of the small room of my office, and to Beth Weinhouse, *Conceive's* editor, who has been the best coach any columnist could want. To my clients, who are a constant source of insight and inspiration. To Gay and Kathlyn Hendricks of the Hendricks Institute for their phenomenal paradigm on the power of connecting the body and the mind. To every friend, and every colleague, every mentor, and every teacher, who has walked some part of this journey with me—you know who you are.

And finally to Linda Parker. Thank you for hobbling into my office, broken foot and all, and opening the door to a whole new world of possibilities. There truly are no accidents.

Author, *Marina Lombardo*

Thank you so much to Kevin Hogan for sharing your wisdom on the human mind, to Elsom Eldridge, Jr. for sharing your expertise, to David Canham for, "dropping everything and taking care of our needs now," to Michele Bryant for your skill and patience in design and layout, and to Debi Fredrick, (wherever you may be) for introducing me to the creativity of Progoff and the unspoken requirement to rock the boat.

My very special thanks go to my family who always supports me through the late nights and tears that accompany every book I write. Thank you Bobby, for finally finding me; thank you Paige for believing in me and sharing your incredible talents in bringing this book to life; and thank you Carson because you are Carson. Finally, I want to thank my mother, Jane Parker, who is living proof that by choice or necessity, great women can and do reinvent themselves through change and growth.

And thank you Marina Lombardo, for being my writing partner and my very treasured friend.

Author, *Linda J. Parker*

Table of Contents

Author's Preface

I first became involved in the field of infertility over ten years ago. Back then, working as a consultant at local fertility centers, facilitating support groups, and designing an educational series for couples about to undergo IVF (in vitro fertilization), I had to scrounge the professional literature to provide guidance that I thought was genuinely meaningful and helpful.

How things have changed!

Now information about the stress of infertility, and the challenges couples face when dealing with it, has hit the mainstream. Turn on a news show or open a magazine and you'll find the latest about the causes, the impact, and the newest fertility treatments. This information explosion has given rise to *Conceive Magazine,* a publication that describes itself as, "the nation's first fertility lifestyle magazine." Within its pages, my column, *Emotionally Speaking,* addresses the unique emotional challenges women can face on the road to creating families.

I practice as a psychotherapist and life coach, in Ocoee, Florida, a small, growing community tucked in a sunshiny corner of southwestern Orlando. There, I work with adults and couples dealing with everyday challenges, as well as the emotional and marital issues that can come with infertility. Over the years, I have realized that the heartache of not being able to conceive touches virtually every area of a woman's life. Infertility affects both how a woman experiences herself and how she relates to her world. But the good news—*and there genuinely is good news*—is that this crisis can serve as a gateway to powerful, positive emotional growth and change.

In my own life, I have also been a student of this process. Striving for a child is an issue that is very close to my heart, and I too, know the feeling of wanting a child so much that I was willing to do almost anything to make that dream come true. Over the years, drawing from my training, my professional work with clients, and of course, my personal experiences, I have developed **seven highly effective tools** for learning from and living through some of life's big challenges. I call these seven powerful, practical, and proven tools (which I share in this book) **an emotional toolbox.**

I want very much to help women and couples facing these issues, arm themselves with their own emotional toolbox of power tools, and reclaim their life. No woman should let her infertility define her. But sometimes knowing how to work through a problem, or even just recognizing the problem to begin with, is more than you can do on your own.

For some readers, *I Am More Than My Infertility, 7 Proven Tools for Turning a Life Crisis into a Personal Breakthrough,* may be all that is needed to help them develop the awareness and skills necessary to restore, rebuild, and reclaim their life. For others, reading this book will be only a starting point. Yet without that critical first step, life remains in deadlock. As the philosopher Lao-Tzu so wisely put it, almost three thousand years ago, *"It is the single small step that begins the journey of a thousand miles."*

While infertility is an issue that affects couples, you will notice this book focuses almost entirely on the challenges and opportunities infertility brings into the lives of women. This book provides answers for the problems of infertility that are unique to women.

Throughout this book I have included stories from my client files, as well as interviews with women whose lives have been changed by infertility. These real life accounts are particularly important because they illustrate both the outcomes that can occur, depending on how each woman chooses to handle her challenges, as well as the power of these transformational tools.

The stories of real women are also important because they serve as tangible evidence that no one walks this path alone. And while knowing this will not necessarily ease the disquiet that weighs so heavily on your heart, it will help empower you with the strength you need to take that first step.

You were an individual of worth and importance before you faced this challenge. You are an individual of worth and importance now. **You are more than your infertility!**

My writing partner, author and educator Linda J. Parker, came to this project from a situation very different from mine. The challenges in her life occurred, not before the conception of a child, but *after*.

Even our writing partnership developed out of something that began as a challenge. While making repairs to her home damaged in 2004 by three hurricanes, (Charley, Frances, and Jean) Linda broke her foot. A conversation between Linda and her doctor, (who happens to be my husband) led the two of us to lunch. Lunch led us to a friendship, a commitment to share with others what we have learned, and the labor of love that ultimately became this book. And if she hadn't broken her foot (or if hurricanes had not damaged her house), Linda and I might never have met!

Most things in life rarely turn out exactly as any of us expect they will, no matter how hard we try to control, coddle, and will them into being the way we envision. We cannot direct the future. We CAN however, prepare ourselves to be strong and flexible, to handle what life hands us, and to do so in ways that enable us to be the individuals of worth and importance we were meant to be. And sometimes, in this transformational process, it becomes possible to create something even bigger than we ever thought was possible for us.

This book was written from training, experience, compassion, and love. This book was written to help you reclaim your life and **turn the life crisis of infertility into a life changing personal breakthrough**.

Be well on your journey!

Marina Lombardo

Foreword by

Dr. Mark Trolice

We are challenged on a daily basis by various scenarios, particularly in our professional and personal lives. Those same challenges and our response mold our personality and enable us to adapt and, ultimately, survive. If we are to succeed in life, we need to learn from our experiences and apply this learning to the next obstacle. But the ability to control our destiny is one of our primal instincts as we struggle to seek our life's purpose.

While it is certainly easy to experience an enriching life with good health, a successful career, and a loving partner, our innate desire to procreate can preoccupy us. As we instinctively attempt to endow our genes, we are at once confronted with our own mortality. The consequence of experiencing difficulty in creating a child can easily convert to an obsession to build a family that may become paralyzing. But why does this compulsion develop and often consume the fertility patient while compelling her to stagnation?

Every patient approaches the step to build a family for a personal reason. For some, there is the love of their partner and desire to bring a child they created to share in their life. Others fear mortality and the loss of their lineage. Yet, most women also have the unique biologic urgency to procreate, however complicated to understand by the male. Nevertheless, if a woman feels any or all of these reasons, then the prospect of infertility is often her first and possibly greatest life crisis. Akin, but in many ways worse than cancer or a chronic pain syndrome, infertility has no cure until holding a child.

Despite loving support of a partner, women perceive infertility as a failure in biologic, sexual, and social terms. Nary can there be a moment that a childless woman is not reminded of her void through family intrusions, friends' invitations to baby birthdays and showers, and the social script portrayed on television. Often, women report their dreams being invaded by their longing for a child. Some cultures place such an importance on childbearing, it is accepted for a man to leave his wife in order to seek a more "fertile" partner. Lastly, the inability to procreate can affect sexual identification and confidence. Unfortunately, this latter aspect is displayed by the potential decreasing amount of intimacy and performance anxiety affecting fertility patients.

Following enough frustration and worry, so begins the repetitive and inconvenience of fertility testing and treatment. Women, albeit anxious, welcome the invasiveness. On the contrary, men often are so private they withdraw from visits and physician recommendations. For the minority, months pass into years of waiting for a positive pregnancy test. The agonizing monthly menses becomes commonplace and a paradoxical indifference and fear of the most aggressive options and alternatives can result.

Time begins to stand still.

How we overcome adversity is the measure of our integrity and character. Our motivation to turn "lemons into lemonade" represents optimism and perseverance. Specifically, the challenge that fertility patients endure results from mourning a life that has not been realized. These patients are described as having their faces pressed up against the windows of families while they long to embrace the dream they do not own. Achievement of their goal may require a new perspective, one that was not originally planned.

For over ten years, I had the unique perspective of being a fertility patient while practicing as a fertility specialist. My passion for the fertility field came first during medical school and has only intensified by my personal struggle. Through years of fertility treatments, my wife and I finally came to closure by adopting our angels. Consequently, I have grown more fervent in assisting others to build their family and in preventing them from becoming consumed in despair. Realizing there are many ways to establish a family, patients have gained hope through the openness of my own challenge.

Seeing firsthand the devastation of fertility couples, I have always firmly believed fertility is a physical, emotional, and financial investment. While the first and third of these commitments are clearly vital, many times the emotional, and spiritual, aspect of a patient's challenge is neglected. Support for this relationship is demonstrated by medical studies showing improved fertility rates following stress reduction as well as acupuncture. As a result, my practice incorporates a full time Reproductive Health Psychologist and Oriental Medical Doctor of Acupuncture. The reason for this it two-fold: pregnancy rates are seemingly higher; and the quality of life for the patient is approached in a positive and healthy way.

In 2004, I approached Marina Lombardo to be on the faculty of our first annual Fertility Awareness Health Fair. Grown from my passion to empower patients and facilitate recognition, my Fertile Dreams Foundation's annual event offers a wide range of lectures from acupuncture and adoption to In-vitro Fertilization and egg donation. Marina graciously volunteered her time and spoke on the topic that became the title of this book. This event inspired Marina to realize her dream and develop an entire guide to assist fertility patients.

As a fellow fertility patient and physician, I can attest to the unique approach Marina gives this topic. *I Am More Than My Infertility: 7 Proven Tools for Turning a Life Crisis into a Personal Breakthrough* encourages enlightenment and personal discovery during an infertility patient's arduous journey of closure and resolve. More than a standard support book, Marina offers hope and the inspiration of "tomorrow" rather than being stagnant in "today."

I applaud Marina's passion toward encouraging efforts of self-fulfillment regardless of the path life may lead us and am confident her book will allow you to grow and overcome this and other challenges. My credo has always been, "the people who face stress and remain healthy thus perceive change not as a threat but as a challenge and sense of opportunity." It has and will always be my privilege to be involved in this aspect of a patient's life as I gain inspiration in watching patients confront and overcome their struggle. Thankfully, we can benefit from the excellent ancillary support such as Marina's to help our patients reach their goals.

Mark P. Trolice, M.D.
Director, Fertility C.A.R.E.
Founder, Fertile Dreams, Inc.

Introduction: A Special Message from

Kim Hahn
Founder of *Conceive Magazine*

It's not a good day when someone informs you that you have no emotional coping skills. But that's exactly what Marina Lombardo told me the first time I met her, more than eight years ago. Even though I was thirty-three years old, had three advanced degrees, earned a very large salary, and had an extremely successful corporate career, apparently I was clueless about how to handle the challenges in my personal life. But spurred by Marina's perception, I embarked on a journey that would change my entire life, including my career. This journey helped me identify and reclaim my own personal power, and gave me the skills to cope with any obstacle that would come my way. The journey was actually the path to finding purpose, joy, peace, love, and gratitude in my life. And Marina Lombardo was by my side, guiding me, for the entire trip.

My first life crisis hit when I was thirty. That's when I was diagnosed with unexplained infertility, after my husband and I had been trying unsuccessfully to get pregnant. It was the first time in my life that I couldn't achieve what I'd set out to do. Throwing money at the problem didn't seem to help, and even after consulting the best fertility doctors in the country, I still wasn't pregnant. After a year and a half of "trying," including one failed IVF (in vitro fertilization) cycle, I found myself in danger of losing everything I'd worked so hard to achieve. I was simply unable to cope.

A friend who was also trying to start a family had started seeing Marina, and highly recommended her. Marina's specialty was helping people who were dealing with infertility, and she knew all the issues and emotions that came with that diagnosis. So I made an appointment, and knew immediately that I'd done the right thing. Marina's style—caring yet direct and honest—was perfect for me.

My first visit with Marina was on July 6, 1999, and exactly one year later—July 6, 2000—I found out I was going to adopt a baby. The year in between was difficult. I tried IVF two more times and failed. I hit bottom, depleted physically, emotionally, and financially. But I also realized during this year that Marina was correct: The reason I was in so much emotional pain was because I didn't have any way of coping with it. And it was during this year that I learned about emotional tools and how to apply them to my life. Thanks to Marina, I learned how to set healthy boundaries in my life (Chapter 5), why telling my truth is so important (Chapter 6,) and how vital it is to take care of my physical health as well as my emotional state (Chapter 3).

Once I started to implement these tools into my personal and professional life, I felt like a kid in a candy store, impatient to use what I was learning to remake my life. I finally realized that I'd never even really wanted to be pregnant. What I wanted was to be a mother, and adoption could make that happen. I'll never forget the day I said goodbye to the fertility specialist. It was such an amazing feeling to recognize that I was finally doing what was absolutely right for me, and only me. I'd spent so much time worrying about what everyone else thought I should do, that I'd almost forgotten who I was and what I wanted. Choosing to adopt my daughter was just the beginning of a process of undoing everything else in my life that I'd only done because I thought it would make other people happy (Chapter 4).

My daughter, Taylor Ann, was born on August 18, 2000, and I was present in the delivery room. Seeing her birth was the most amazing experience of my life, and it unleashed something in me that made me want to possess even more of this power I'd claimed in order to become a mother. Now I wanted to go even further in creating the life I wanted to live. Marina told me that the best gift anyone can give a child is a healthy mother and father. When Taylor's biological mother handed me her child, I knew that now I had to be the best parent I could possibly be. So I began a mission—with Marina's help—to be as emotionally and physically healthy as I could be, and to create for myself a "life without limits."

My daughter is seven years old now, and I still practice using the tools Marina has shown me. I've applied these tools to every aspect of my life. I've been able to face and heal the pain of childhood trauma, start my own company, improve my marriage and relationships, and live a life with meaning and purpose. Most of all, I have given my daughter a healthy mother who can raise her to be the person she is meant to be.

Marina's blunt comment to me that first day, telling me that I didn't have any emotional coping skills, gave me the opportunity to change my life before it was too late. Without that intervention, it would have taken me a lot longer to recognize my unhappiness, and I would have had many more things in my past to undo. In a way I was fortunate that my crisis happened when I was still relatively young.

At age thirty-seven, I found the courage and strength to leave my lucrative corporate career to start an award-winning publication, *Conceive Magazine*, for women who want information about starting a family. I didn't want any woman to have to suffer as much as I had, without consumer-friendly and reliable information about baby-making. In the past few years my company has grown to include *Conceive On-Air* (an internet radio series), ConceiveOnLine.com, and a new series of fertility books.

Infertility is only one of a number of life crises that can strike any of us. The key to surviving a crisis—and even thriving—is to be open to the life lessons that are there to learn. By incorporating the tools that Marina lays out in this book, you'll be able to approach all of your life challenges with a sense of confidence, hope, and gratitude.

Thank you, Marina. I couldn't have done it without you. I will always be grateful to you for telling me I had no emotional coping skills...and then helping me to develop the good, strong tools I'm equipped with now. It was those tools, and your support, that helped me find the courage to adopt my daughter and to change my life. I know that with this book, you will be able to bring your message to an even larger audience, and help others find the emotional tools they need to handle life's challenges.

Kim Hahn
Founder and CEO
Conceive Magazine, Inc.

Instructions for

How to Read this Book

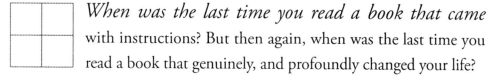 *When was the last time you read a book that came* with instructions? But then again, when was the last time you read a book that genuinely, and profoundly changed your life?

I Am More Than My Infertility, 7 Proven Tools for Turning a Life Crisis into a Personal Breakthrough, is life changing, but in order for you to experience the effect of all the book has to offer, you have do more than just read the words that are written on the pages.

Read this book and be open to receive the powerful healing message it brings. Read this book because you are ready to become a stronger woman and because you just want to feel peace, happiness, and hope again.

And as you read this book, be sure you:

- Give yourself permission to read *slowly*. This is not a romance novel that you curl up with on a rainy Sunday afternoon and read from start to finish. This is a real world, *life process*. Read a chapter, or even a few pages, and then set the book aside and process into your own life and your own emotions what you have read.

- Accept that this book is about change and while change is often a good thing, it can also be stressful in and of itself. Work to keep your mind open to the messages of this book, and receptive to the truths—even the painful to hear ones—that it holds.

- Practice the tools and techniques you are learning. Each chapter comes with examples, exercises, and lots of new ideas. Don't wait until you have read the final chapter to begin implementing them. Statistics[1] show if you attend a conference and you do not begin to incorporate into your life the things you have learned at the conference within three days of leaving it, you are not ever likely to use the tools you have probably spent several days studying. In the same way, the tools of this book require that you commit to trying them; and discipline yourself to making them part of your life, and that most importantly, you do it NOW, while you are immersed in the book.

- Keep the book by your bedside, in your bag, or other convenient place so that you can read it in small bites, and re-read the parts that you find especially helpful or especially challenging. Turning a life crisis into a personal breakthrough isn't an overnight experience and your progress will come in stages with plateaus and even times when you move backward instead of forward. Accept that this is okay; simply give yourself permission to be yourself.

There's More:

The *I Am More Than My Infertility Personal Breakthrough Tool Kit* is available as a downloadable program or in CD format at **www.IAmMore.net** or **www.MarinaLombardo.com** to help you take the 7 proven tools to a deeper, more personal level of use as you turn the life crisis of infertility into your own breakthrough. The Tool Kit is your companion as you begin, from wherever you are, to move toward peace and clarity, and create the fulfilling, satisfying life you deserve.

---

[1] Cloud, Henry "Action Steps for Monday" speech at the 2005 Willow Creek Association Leadership Summit. Barrington, Illinois, August 11—13, 2005.

Throughout this book, you will find many stories
from the lives of real women and their personal struggles
with the issues of fertility. All of their names,
as well as any telltale specifics about their personal lives,
have been changed to protect their privacy.
The facts of their experiences are presented just as they occurred.

You Are
More Than...

Michelle Bloom and Jan Kettering are two women— perhaps very much like you—who know all too well what it means to face the challenges of fertility. Attractive, thirty-ish, both have careers they enjoy, happy marriages, and homes in neighborhoods only a few blocks apart.

Although they live near one another, their paths never crossed until each of them turned to a local fertility specialist for treatment. One moment they were strangers and the next, they were oddly connected by a life crisis for which neither of them was prepared.

Then five years passed and Michelle and Jan did not see each other—not until a Thursday night meeting of the local chapter of RESOLVE.[2] Jan Kettering was the guest speaker, and making presentations to a group always left her a little nervous and preoccupied. When the meeting broke for coffee and sodas, she found her first chance to really look around the room. One of the group's organizers, a tall woman with a long blonde ponytail,

[2] RESOLVE. The National Infertility Association. See website http://www.resolve.org/

caught her eye. For a moment, Jan couldn't place her and then a familiar flip of the ponytail triggered her memory. Jan knew it had to be Michelle.

"Do you remember me?"

Michelle's thin face filled with her warm smile. "Of course I do. I was hoping to get a chance to talk to you and wondering if you'd remember all the hours you and I spent sitting in Dr. Bailey's waiting room. We were there at the same time so often I used to think the scheduling nurse planned it that way. How in the world are you?"

"Great!" Then Jan hesitated. It *had* been a long time. What if Michelle was still seeing Dr. Bailey?

Michelle waved one hand casually as she spoke, "These days, the only waiting room I frequent is at the pediatrician's office. My son was born three and a half years ago, after my second IVF."

"Oh Michelle, that's wonderful! And I have a beautiful daughter named Courtney, who we adopted almost four years ago."

"Jan, I am so happy for you and just think, after all our heartbreak, we both have children now. But why are you conducting seminars on infertility—weren't you in human resources at a pharmaceutical company, or something like that?"

Jan smiled. "Funny isn't it? As I worked through my personal struggle, I became aware of how profoundly infertility changed my life. I learned a lot about how I perceive myself. After talking to other women, I realized I wasn't alone in my experience. So I took my career in a whole new direction. I just love what I am doing now."

"Who would have thought five years ago that our lives would turn out like this…but tell me," Michelle lowered her voice as she leaned in closer, "don't you still feel angry every time you see a pregnant woman?"

Jan poured a cup of coffee and slowly stirred sugar into her cup. "No," she said honestly, "I no longer feel angry about it at all."

First You Get Mad

Michelle and Jan's story represents two very different ways of handling the life crisis of infertility. Most women who face issues of fertility feel anger— at least for a while. It's hard not to feel angry or resentful when pregnancy is not easy for you, yet seems to be so simple for your friends, your sister, and all those smiling women in maternity clothes that you see in restaurants and shopping malls. Michelle and Jan both experienced the anger that is a natural part of dealing with infertility, along with the sadness, guilt, bitterness, shame, confusion, and frustration that come from trying without success to conceive a child. But, it is at this critical point where the similarities between Michelle and Jan end.

Modern science and age-old wisdom both offer many approaches that may lead to the conception of a child. Adoption offers other alternatives for building families. Although the presence of a child ends your state of childlessness, it does not heal the wounds of infertility. Like other types of life crises, infertility challenges you to look closely at yourself and your way of functioning in the world. Infertility, and the stress that comes with it, brings to the surface parts of you that need to heal and grow. If you don't address these issues, and a child enters your life, you resolve only one aspect of the situation, but none of the others. The problems that surface before a baby arrives do not go away, even though your joy at having a child may temporarily overshadow them. Quite simply, if you ignore the invitation of this challenge, not even the birth of a beautiful child allows you to emerge whole. In this regard, the baby is neither the prize, nor the solution.

For Jan, the trauma of infertility served as an impetus to a period of

⊞ *although the presence of a child ends your state of childlessness, it does not heal the wounds of infertility*

intense self-evaluation. She began to see that her struggles with infertility revealed deficiencies in her coping skills that had been there all along. Under the pressures of trying to battle her own biology, other unresolved issues became more obvious. Old wounds and past problems surfaced because they were now the backdrop for the new issue she faced. When Jan opened the door to address her new challenges, baggage she had never unpacked, came tumbling down on top of her.

You may understand firsthand what it feels like to be optimistically moving through life, expecting each month to be "the month". Suddenly, without even the warning of caution signs and blinking lights to alert you, you come face to face with a leviathan parked in your path.

Uninvited and unwelcome, infertility and all of its issues move into your life; so pervasive it can easily establish itself as the center of your world. Fertility issues work their way into every nook and cranny until eventually, you view your entire life through the lens of your infertility. Fertility problems quickly build a massive, frightening, and wearisome barrier, stealing momentum and bringing life plans to a halt. Your options become surprisingly limited.

When fertility challenges create such a barricade, you have very few choices. You can screech to a halt, cowering behind this obstacle in depression and self-blame. You can beat your head against it in frustration. Or you can do what Jan did. You can find a way to dismantle the barrier, brick by brick.

Jan could not change the fact that an obstacle blocked her from going where she wanted to go. But she could create a plan for managing her challenges in positive and productive ways. Jan could take down enough bricks to enable her to get over the obstacle and eventually, move beyond it.

Dealing with both the new and the old issues in Jan's life was as much hard work as if she had literally rolled up her sleeves and manually disman-tled a wall of bricks and mortar. She had to face the new emotions inherent in her fertility struggle, while at the same time, coming to terms with old issues as they surfaced. She had to do it without blaming all of her anger and sadness on her difficulties conceiving a child—that would have been an easy out, but it wouldn't have been honest and it wouldn't have made her the resilient individual she ultimately became.

Instead, Jan tackled her problem head on and used her situation as an opportunity to grow. Her efforts helped her become more self-aware. She learned to communicate her feelings and her needs more effectively. She became better at setting personal boundaries. As time went on, not only did Jan's relationships with others improve, so did her sense of self-worth. As a different, stronger woman than she had been before, she changed ca-reers to one she found more satisfying, and she created a lifestyle that truly reflected the new person she had become. After grieving the realization that she would not be able to have a biological child, Jan embraced the op-portunity for adoption. She moved beyond seeing herself as a woman de-fined by infertility and she welcomed a new phase in her life.

Depending upon your personal coping skills and your stage in your fertility challenge, you may find it difficult at this time to iden-tify with Jan. You may find it hard to see that anything positive could ever come from this unwanted turn in your life. At first, Jan felt this way, too. Yet, with time, she found she was actually grateful for the growth and the changes her struggle brought into her life. As you personally experience the overwhelming issues of fertility, try to leave the door open—even if it is just a crack—for the possibility that someday you too can live your own version of Jan's story.

In contrast to Jan's proactive approach, when Michelle hit the brick wall, she did not attempt to back up, get a running start, and scale it. She didn't even try to dismantle it slowly. Instead, she let it close in around her. Despite the fact that Michelle achieved a successful pregnancy, part of her remained stuck in her grief. She did not use her experience as an opportunity for personal growth. Even though Michelle gave birth to a beautiful, healthy biological child, in many ways, she remained bitter that she had to undergo the infertility experience at all. She defined her life and her purpose by her fertility or lack of it, when in fact Michelle was much, much more.

Many women face their infertility believing that if they can only have a child, all of their problems will go away. But infertility isn't resolved because of a pregnancy or an adoption. A baby never really "fixes" anything and Michelle, along with thousands of other women like her, are living proof that, if you let it, infertility will compromise or even destroy the quality of life you could be enjoying.

Even though you may believe something precious has been taken from you, you still have choices. You can do nothing at all and risk winding up like Michelle. You'll be flat lining on the emotional growth chart, wrapped in the burden of your own unresolved grief.

Or you can take this book and do what Jan did. Use these powerful life tools to help you start, wherever you are now, and move forward, achieving as much personal growth as possible.

confusion precedes growth

You are so much more than your infertility. Pick up your toolbox and make the promise to yourself that you are going to use this challenge as an opportunity to become a stronger, more empowered woman. With this goal ahead of you, you are ready to examine the tools you need in your emotional toolbox in order to achieve this change and growth.

Stress Happens

Here are two irrefutable facts. First, and above all else, fertility issues create stress. Second, stress impacts your body, and very often, your fertility, too. Yet, what you may not realize is that having the right tools in your emotional toolbox—and using those tools—is your most effective means of dealing with this stress. Look more closely at this connection.

Everyone is familiar with that stressed out feeling. Deadlines to meet; sitting in traffic unable to make meetings or scheduled appointments; too much on your plate and too few hours in the day. During times of stress, your body responds by exhibiting the classic "fight or flight" response. You probably have heard of this and perhaps you even recognize it when it happens to you.

When your body is in the fight or flight mode, your heart beats faster, you breathe more rapidly, and your muscles tense. Your body releases stress hormones. Over time, if stressful demands continue to barrage your body, the on-going release of stress hormones compromises your immune system. In a perfect world, you would have downtime after a stressful situation, so your body could recover and return to normal. *But when was the last time you lived in a perfect world?*

The stress of infertility is especially unique because it is cyclical and ongoing. Nature doesn't allow for much-needed downtime. Your stress level soars as you fluctuate between the high anticipation that this time things will work out, to the crushing disappointment of a failed procedure. When you add fertility treatment, with its medical procedures, potent drugs, expense, and high demands for involvement and compliance, you could very well be mixing the formula for your own personal toxic cocktail of emotions. The ingredients list can include invasive procedures; your already strained relationships with spouse, friends, and family; that juggling act you regularly perform between your job and your other responsibilities; all those feelings of anxiety and failure; and of course, those unwanted menstrual periods that come each month. Under these conditions, your body just cannot get the bounce back time it requires to heal and restore itself. The price you pay is both psychological *and* physical exhaustion.

the stress of infertility is unique because it is cyclical and ongoing

In the simplest terms, learning to manage both your stress and your life with the help of this emotional toolbox makes good common sense. Not only will these seven emotional tools help you feel better, they will allow you to grow beyond what you thought was possible. You will pay down the emotional debt that has been accumulating and you will prevent new charges from piling up. Even if you are not motivated to deal with your stress for your own benefit, or for your marriage, research has shown that there is a definitive relationship between fertility and stress.

"Although it's not the only factor, there is clear evidence that stress can interfere with conception," says Machelle Seibel, M.D., professor of obstetrics and gynecology at the University of Massachusetts Medical School in Worcester, and a prominent researcher in the field. "When women learn to control their stress with relaxation techniques, their rates of anxiety and depression go down, and their rates of conception go up, although they might still need medical help."[3]

---

[3] Kalish, Nancy. *Conceive Magazine*, "Fertility Retreats," Spring 2005, p.23.

Life Crisis Number One

Infertility is not only stressful; it also meets the criteria for being a life crisis. In the realm of crises, infertility is often one of the first for many women, and even more often, the very first crisis a married couple faces together. A crisis occurs when something overwhelming happens for which you do not feel prepared. A characteristic of a crisis is that you do not have adequate coping skills, or the skills you have do not sufficiently equip you for what you are facing.

One young couple in particular, serves as a classic example. Newly married, neither one had ever learned to deal with conflict. When arguments occurred, they would simply go to bed and the next day, act as if nothing had happened. That was fine early in their relationship, when the issues they were dealing with were small and easier to brush under the rug. But when they hit the infertility wall, their method of coping broke down—it did not serve their needs. They had to learn to communicate effectively in order to make decisions together.

In essence, a life crisis is an opportunity to evolve beyond what you thought was possible for you. A crisis is a catalyst for growth. As you read this, you may be thinking, "Please spare me the cliché that all things happen for a reason." That's not the message here. Honestly, no one knows why some things happen. You may live your lifetime and never be able to come up with one good reason why infertility happened to you. There are couples who are never able to have children, yet would be the most ideal parents imaginable. And as unfair as it seems, other couples, who shouldn't even have a license to drive a car, seem to have children effortlessly. But the bottom line is this: *it is what it is.*

a crisis is a catalyst for growth

Infertility, like so many things in life, is not based on fairness, individual merit, or logic. Whether or not you have a medical diagnosis, you will probably never have a good reason to explain *why* this has happened to you.

For whatever reason, life itself is not fair. Unjust, unconscionable things happen every day—with no recognizable rhyme or reason. Unfortunately, no one walks through life without being dealt some misfortune. There is an old adage that says, if you walked into a crowded room and every person put their troubles in the middle of the room with the option to keep their own or trade for the problems of someone else, most people would look at the reality of other people's lives and then walk away, taking back their own troubles.

It is what it is.

You don't need to hear sappy advice about keeping your chin up, or looking on the bright side. However, you do need to understand that you have choices. Whether you emerge whole or broken from your fertility challenge is up to you. You have within you everything you need to learn the skills to help you thrive now, and live healthier and happier for the rest of your life. You can learn to talk to your spouse or partner in a way that truly works and you can have a stronger, closer partnership to show for it. If you embrace this process, you must move toward rather than away from the pain of it. You can do this only if you first arm yourself with the power tools you need to work your way through your issues.

Seven essential power tools make up your emotional toolbox. Imagine them like a pyramid, with each skill forming the foundation for building the next skill. These power tools are:

1. Take care of your body.

Taking care of *you* is the most fundamental and powerful of all the tools. It is also the one over which you have the most control. Ironically, it can be the most challenging because *of how you may be experiencing yourself emotionally.* Your fertility struggles may have resulted in you feeling angry with your body, as if your body is betraying you. Self-anger or self-loathing makes caring for yourself a challenge. Learning to nurture your body, and recognizing that your body is doing the best it can, are realizations that will genuinely transform you.

2. Make conscious choices.

Making conscious choices is a life skill that should always be firmly in place, but the demands of infertility make it essential for you to make choices in which YOU are the top priority. If you are like many women, you already struggle with this; you make everyone else's needs and feelings more important than your own. NOW is the time to learn how to *check in* with yourself, and to make choices that are right for you.

3. Set healthy boundaries.

Healthy boundaries mean learning to care for yourself *while* you are in relationships with other people. Healthy boundaries are an extension of the conscious choices you make—you learn to check in with yourself, and then to structure your relationships with others to respect what you have chosen. In order for your relationships with others to work well, learning to take healthy responsibility for yourself, and allowing others to do the same, is vital.

4.   Tell the truth.

An essential component of making conscious choices and setting healthy boundaries, telling the truth is a tool that addresses the language you use to communicate to yourself and to those around you. The "truth" tool teaches you how to discover and speak *your own* truth and how to let go of the punishing lies that are part of negative self-talk. Just as importantly, it teaches you how to use effective language in relationships, especially the most intimate ones, where there's the temptation to pretend not to know the very things about which you need to be talking!

5.   Take quiet space.

The need for quiet space is two-fold. On one hand, the demands of infertility and its treatment, places squarely on your lap, an overload of information you must decipher in order to make important medical decisions. On the other hand, the mere existence of infertility in your life calls you to reconsider how you perceive yourself, how you care for yourself, and how you care for those around you. This tool teaches you how to create quiet space in your day so you can restore your spirit and discover the wisdom of your own inner guidance.

6.   Give yourself permission to grieve.

Grief is an inevitable part of infertility, from the initial diagnosis to the cycles of hope and despair that surround each failed procedure. Within the quiet space you take, it is essential to take the time you need to grieve.

Grieving honors the diverse range of emotions that infertility brings with it. Healthy grief means you come to see these emotions as sacred, rather than as inconvenient. Learning the skill of becoming your own companion on this leg of the journey is key. Realizing you are not alone, and that there is healing in the loving support of fellow travelers, is equally as important. Grief is the gateway through which you must pass as you journey to hope, to healing, and eventually, to acceptance.

7.   See the big picture.

When your world becomes all about your infertility, it is hard to recall what your life was like before, and it may feel like your situation will go on forever. But if you know how to step out of the situation, even just a bit, and then know what to look for and how to ask, *miracles can and DO happen.* Like diamonds in the rough, hidden within these very challenges are often gifts—opportunities, people, information, and circumstances—that have the power to transform your life in ways, which right now, may be hard to imagine.

So get ready. The tools you are about to discover truly have the power to change the rest of your life...

The Power Tools for Your Journey

You wouldn't think of going on a trip without packing the right clothing, would you? In much the same way, you also have to pack a toolbox of the right power tools to help you on your journey through life. But no matter how transformational these tools are, (and they truly *are*) they only have value when you choose to use them in your life in a practical way.

The skill-building exercises in this book help you do just that. At the end of every chapter, you will find a page designed to help you apply the ideas of the chapter to your own life. Specifically, these exercises help you take the wisdom and tools from these pages and put them to work for you. Each exercise shows you the way to "plug in" your tools, power them up, and get to work.

So get a notebook or journal, and get ready to use the power tools to rewrite this chapter of your life.

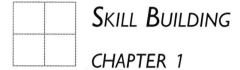

SKILL BUILDING

CHAPTER 1

1. Reread the story of Jan and Michelle. With whom do you honestly identify?
   Are you more like Jan or more like Michelle? Why?

2. What areas of your life give evidence to you being a "Jan"? Which ones
   show you are being a "Michelle"?

3. If you find yourself more like Michelle, what has been the fallout from some
   of your choices? Are you ready to make a change?

4. Look at the list of power tools:

   Take Care of Your Body

   Make Conscious Choices

   Set Healthy Boundaries

   Tell the Truth

   Take Quiet Space

   Give Yourself Permission to Grieve

   See the Big Picture

   Which of the seven do you already feel you have under control?

   Which ones represent a place where you feel stuck?

The First Crisis of Your Marriage

You know what they say, "...it's the journey, not the destination." This is one of those frustrating but perceptively accurate insights into life. If only life was about hitting a target, your existence could be predictable and orderly. You would marathon through certain stages and then enjoy the fruits of your labor—your perfect destination realized. Of course, life never works this way. And the wisdom of understanding that life is all about the journey applies to the issues of fertility perhaps more profoundly than to any other experience you may ever face.

Most women are only in the first leg of their life excursion when infertility so frustratingly fixes itself as an obstacle in their paths. Often times, they are in that first flush of solidifying their identities as an adult—developing careers, relationships, and homes with the objective of having these things neatly in place before they start building a family. More importantly, at the point most women initially face infertility, they are not only in the critical developmental stages of adulthood, they are usually in the early developmental stages of their marriage or partnership. Infertility is frequently the first life crisis a couple faces together.

Testing Your Wedding Vows

When you stood at the altar, aglow in wedding day bliss, you made a vow to love, honor, and cherish, "for better or worse…in sickness and in health." Who knew it should have included the caveats, "even when I am bouncing off the wall from the effects of fertility medications," or "despite the fact that we feel heartbroken and desolate over the child we cannot have"?

Whatever you planned for your life's journey together, it didn't involve testing your relationship with the intense emotional strain that accompanies fertility problems. Whatever you planned, *it just wasn't this.*

Infertility, so often the first personal crisis of a marriage, is a complex issue for couples. First, there are the mental and physical stresses that are inherent in the treatments themselves, and then there are the financial concerns, and the difficulty in knowing when to go on and when to give up. Chapters 3, 4, 5, and 6, which talk about the first four power tools, give you important insights and effective strategies to deal with these aspects of your journey. Fertility challenges also bring an unparalleled sense of disappointment and loss, which sadly is intrinsic to the very diagnosis of infertility. The fifth and sixth power tools, presented in chapters 7 and 8, help you work through the overwhelming emotions you may experience.

Right now, however, you must first address the tensions that can occur in your relationship simply because fertility issues affect men and women in such significantly different ways. Within the stressors that occur because of this, you have a choice—some couples experience monumental growth as a result of living through this crisis together. Jan Kettering and her husband Michael are one of those couples.

"Michael and I always had a good marriage," Jan related, "but looking back now, I see how we'd skirt over some issues, and try to avoid talking about the uncomfortable stuff. When infertility hit, we were blindsided. For the first time, we had to learn to talk

no matter what is happening in your life, you need to make a conscious effort to grow your relationship

to each other; I mean *really* talk, about the hard stuff. And there were so many times when we felt as if we had only each other to turn to, so we had to learn to be there for each other like never before. All of it made our love stronger somehow, and now we have what so many couples our age don't have—the awareness that no matter how tough things get, we can count on each other to be there." Then she paused, looked away for a moment, and continued, "But the getting there…well, that part wasn't always easy."

The experience of infertility is often a turning point, or crisis, in the life of a couple. The Chinese written language has a hanzi or symbol for the concept of crisis. In its simplest translation, this symbol contains the elements of both danger and opportunity. The universal language of infertility could easily include such a symbol, because danger and opportunity coexist within this challenge. The danger innate in infertility includes stress, financial concerns, and most importantly, the risks of potentially having to re-envision or reinvent your life in a way you never imagined. Nevertheless, within fertility's danger lies the enormous opportunity for couples to flourish in their love for one another. Utilizing your exceptional opportunity starts with personal growth and mutual understanding. To achieve such growth in your marriage, you must first understand the tremendous differences in how men and women process infertility.

Yours and Mine

Since infertility is a problem you and your husband or partner experience together, *why is it so different for each of you, and why do you deal with it in such different ways?*

Quite simply, when it comes to infertility, you and your husband have extremely different perspectives. These differences are apparent in more than just the unique ways any two people might handle the same problem. The struggle for you to become a mother is a vastly different process than the struggle for your husband to become a father.

Besides the obvious gender differences, expectations in today's world are different for you than they are for your husband. As much as women have opportunities today as never before, if you are like many other women, no matter what else you accomplish, becoming a mother is still truly important in your life. Being a mother is a primary way women bond to one another, in much the same way that careers or sports are ways many men build bonds. When you become a mother, you develop a special connection to other women who have shared the motherhood experience.

Moreover, the social conditioning that defines the roles of parents is vastly different for each gender. You and your spouse or partner approach parenthood with certain preconceived ideas about which responsibilities of parenting belong to the father and which ones belong to the mother. While your own ideas of motherhood may be traditional or nontraditional, they still represent a "script" that you feel expected to follow. Such scripts are deeply ingrained, and are the result of your upbringing within your family and your perception of what you believe society expects from you.

To help you better understand how strong internal definitions of motherhood and fatherhood really are, for the moment, forget your own feelings about struggling to become a mother. Instead, try to imagine what you would feel if your role were one of struggling to become a father.

Difficult to imagine, isn't it?

When you try to view your circumstances from your spouse's perspective, it quickly becomes apparent that you and your husband are reacting very differently to the experience you are sharing. Typically, the woman carries the greatest burden of infertility—even when the actual cause is undiagnosed, or even when the cause has to do with the husband.

Perhaps you feel guilty about your inability to conceive, imagining that you are depriving your husband of a child and your parents of a grandchild. Whether or not this loss is one your spouse and other family members actually experience does not matter. The fact that you *perceive* it exists, is sufficient for it to become a great source of guilt and anxiety in your life.

There are also differences in how infertility is experienced within the marital relationship itself. In general, women tend to focus on their personal struggle of wanting a baby. Men may focus more on the impact infertility struggles have on their wives, and on the marriage. Men, perceiving the struggle their wives are experiencing, have a deep desire to find a way to remedy the situation and get life, and their wives, back on track. Wives, on the other hand, often simply want their husbands to listen to them and to support them emotionally during their struggle. These are significant differences in coping styles, and this, more than any other single factor, is where many relationship troubles begin.

In fact, you and your husband do not think or even speak about the challenges of fertility, using the same words. Considering how different your perspectives are, what do you think are the odds that both you and your spouse or partner will have exactly the same feelings about which, if any, fertility treatments are best to try, and for how long, and at what cost?

Obviously, your reactions and those of your husband are not going to be the same.

Men traditionally want to "fix" problems. When they can't fix the problem, frustration directed at themselves inevitably spills over onto their spouse. You've seen this happen before with small issues. You tell your husband that the air conditioner in your car/the stopper in the bathroom sink/ or the password on your credit card account is not working and he tries to resolve the trouble. If he succeeds, he's happy, you're happy, and life goes forward without problems. However, if he fails, he is annoyed at himself and at the car/sink/or computer for not being more "fixable". He's not going to yell at himself, and it is not very satisfying to yell at the bathroom sink, so he yells at you—after all, you brought this problem to light. If he isn't a shouter, then he may just slam the door, or detach himself from a situation he finds frustrating.

Do all men handle problems they don't know how to address by getting angry or by withdrawing? Of course not, but many men do, at least to some degree. When your spouse sees your sadness and pain, *because he loves you,* he wants to fix the problem. But infertility is one problem that may defy his best efforts to fix. In as much as a woman may feel she is failing the marriage by not conceiving, a man is likely to feel as if he is failing his wife by not having a solution for this problem.

Your husband feels his own pain over the struggle the two of you are experiencing, and he feels disappointment in himself that he cannot make things right for you and for your marriage. Remembering this can help you understand his responses and then make better choices about how you react to things he says, does, or fails to say and do.

Your husband will not always respond the way you want him to whether the issue is fertility or anything else you may face together. However, if he really is as wonderful as you thought he was the day you said, "I do," then it helps to keep in mind that he is not necessarily doing the wrong thing, because he is insensitive or unloving. Sometimes he does the wrong thing because the way he's wired, and has been conditioned, is just plain different from your wiring and your conditioning. Sometimes, he does the wrong thing for the same reason you do—he just can't figure out what **your** right thing is.

You Are In This Together

You and your husband may someday have a child together but you will never erase the infertility experience the two of you are sharing. Once again, *it is what it is,* and this is as true for you as a couple as it is for you as an individual.

But within this challenge is an amazing opportunity. Together you can use this experience like Jan and Michael did, to build incredible bonds of intimacy and strength—to help you grow a rock-solid marriage. Or you can let the wrong behaviors take hold and turn a potentially good marriage into something miserable for both of you.

When you and your husband fail to acknowledge these differences, it gets easy for you to become polarized, each of you feeling as if the other cannot empathize with you or understand your feelings. As a result, when you and your husband face this dilemma, you can quickly fall into a number of relationship-damaging behaviors.

You can fight about your situation. You can each blame the other person. You can lose yourself in busyness or work. You can sweep touchy subjects under the rug. Ultimately, you can even let this situation destroy your marriage. But whatever you do during this—the first crisis of your

it is what it is

marriage—you need to be very aware that you are setting in motion powerful patterns of interaction. Once these patterns are in place, they quickly ingrain themselves in the marriage and become default behaviors for both of you. How you as a couple handle the crisis of infertility has lifelong impact and defines how you deal with any major problem that occurs during your years together.

Stand back and look at what is going on in your lives. Whether you are undergoing fertility treatment or taking a less aggressive approach to conception, together you and your husband are still investing your time, your emotions, your hard earned money, and a substantial chunk of your spirits into your efforts to give birth to a child. You are each doing this, hopefully because you want to enrich your future lives together with a child who is uniquely yours. Whether it happens or not, recognize how much love and devotion to each other and to the marriage is required for you to be making this effort together. You clearly have a very special relationship and this alone is worthy of nurturing. Every time the stresses of infertility leave you frustrated with your husband or your marriage, go back to this moment and reaffirm: *we must love each other a lot to go through this.*

Building Bridges

Couples confronting fertility problems have a remarkable opportunity to get ahead in the marriage game, to grow as a couple and as a team. This period of stress can also be a time of building bridges above the dangers and traumas that show up in your life and pose a threat to your relationship. You and your husband can build a mutually supportive structure that connects you with each other, and with your bright future on the other side.

The first important step in building such bridges has less to do with talking to your partner and more to do with your internal dialogue. Be on the lookout for self-talk that puts an unfair, negative spin on you and your relationship. Disarm this enemy by confronting him and shining the light of truth on the leviathan that sits in your path. Like a monster you feared in your childhood closet, once you drag your fears out into the open, you will discover that they are far less menacing than you imagined.

When you think about your situation, look realistically at the possibilities. Because many women do not actually acknowledge to themselves or ever say aloud how stigmatized they feel by their struggle, "the unspoken" of infertility lurks silently in the dark, empowered by its own concealment. Unfortunately, these feelings of grief cannot help but spill over into the marital relationship.

Being honest with yourself about the burden you are carrying and the lies you are telling yourself, makes it much easier for you and your spouse or partner to talk to each other. Just being able to say aloud, "I am afraid you will not love me as much if I can't have a child," or "I am embarrassed that people will think we did not try hard enough if we stop the treatments now," can be a tremendous relief to you. Once these thoughts and feelings are out in the open, where you and your husband can discuss them, neither of you will have to fear any longer that the undercurrent of this negativity will be acted out and undermine your relationship. You have drawn a line beyond which the leviathan cannot go any farther; you have set a cap on the monster's perceived powers. Keep in mind, you are not facing this alone; you and your husband have the beast outnumbered two to one.

Think about the list of reasons you were first attracted to this man in your life—smart, funny, kind—but chances are, "mind reader" was not on the list. Sometimes you develop the attitude that if your spouse really loves you, he will "just know" how you feel. *How unrealistic!* Life is complicated enough; don't expect your husband to jump through hoops that include

couples confronting fertility problems have a remarkable opportunity to get ahead in the marriage game

becoming a psychic intuitive. Every time you choose to take a breath, to be honest with yourself about your feelings, and then to communicate them just as candidly to your husband, you are dragging that leviathan out into the bright light of day and acknowledging your challenges for what they are. When you step forward boldly and do this, you will be amazed at how your monster begins to whither and shrink under the scrutiny of truthfulness and the power of a loving, supportive marriage.

As you and your husband talk, try to become aware of your own patterns and default behaviors. For example, if you want to discuss something with your husband, but the TV distracts him, how do you react? Do you tend to silently sulk and walk away, freezing him out, even when he asks you, "what's wrong?" Do you indirectly communicate what you need, hoping he will pick up the cues? Do you become extremely busy, and avoid personal interaction, in a fruitless effort to manage your anxiety? These reactions are not exclusive to your infertility struggle—they were probably around long before now. Nevertheless, you can be sure that if these are your default behaviors during times of stress, they will rear their heads during the stress of infertility.

You are in a critical stage of your life, dealing with life-defining issues. The cost of falling back on your old patterns, or of creating destructive new ones, can be particularly high. Now more than ever, you need to find ways to move beyond these behaviors and to talk directly about what you need and how you feel.

Ask questions rather than presuming you already know how he feels. Making assumptions about your husband can be a disastrous error. Try not to assume you know what your spouse or partner is thinking and feeling. If he is not talking to you for whatever reason, don't attempt to guess or assign emotions to him that may not be correct. Instead, in a neutral way, just tell him what you notice, or what you think you understand.

For example, you could assume your husband's silence means he is bored with all the discussions of fertility treatment and does not care what you try next, or if you ever get pregnant. However, if jumping to conclusions is one of your default behaviors, look out! Instead of making assumptions, try asking him how he feels by saying something like, "I noticed you were very quiet at the doctor's office today. What did you think about his suggestions?" Or, "How is all this for you?"

As he speaks, really listen to the words he says, and pay attention to the things he leaves unsaid. Remember, the goal is to understand one another—not to agree on everything.

Be aware also of the need to address issues as they arise. If you start to notice that you are overreacting to little irritations or minor annoyances, look out for the leviathan lurking beneath the surface. Take the time to think about whether the un-replaced roll of toilet paper is really what's irking you, or whether there's something bigger on your mind.

Creating Balance

Infertility, if you let it, will be a dilemma that insidiously permeates every corner of your marriage until eventually there is nothing else left. You must create a balance where you give this issue its due *and* you proactively make time for other aspects of your life.

Even if you and your husband are a couple who can talk easily about your infertility challenges, you do not want this topic to find its way into every conversation you have. Instead, give yourself a preset time when you will talk about your current issues of fertility and then stick to your schedule. For instance, you might set aside some time each evening to talk. Be sure to pick a time when you are both free from distractions, and make a pact not to answer the telephone during this time. One idea that fills this criterion, (as well as has an added bonus of exercise) is to go for a walk together after supper, and make that your time to talk. When the agreed upon time is up, stop talking. Then make time to be about other things, as individuals and as a couple. As you put the topic away, feel the relief of draping a tarpaulin over the monster now snoring in your pathway, and it *will* be snoring, because it won't find your calm and rational discussions nearly as interesting as you do.

Putting the subject of infertility in its proper place allows you to create time for the rest of your life. Imagine drawing a circle around your relationship, and then allowing the subject of infertility inside the circle only during specified times. Creating this type of private oasis within your marriage, and having times when infertility lives outside the circle, allows you to be open to the possibility of other issues and other interests.

Spend time talking to your husband about ways to nurture one another and the relationship. Think back to when you first started dating and recall some of the things you loved to do. Buying an annual pass to something you both enjoy, like theatre, or a theme park, can ensure that you always have something fun on tap. Be sure to put time aside for these dates, rather than leaving things to chance. The best intentions go down the drain without a commitment. Schedule your time together, as you would anything else that is a priority in your life.

This is also a good time to consider taking on some new hobbies, such as ballroom dancing, playing golf, or training together at the gym. Such activities are wonderful because they can connect you to each other in a *positive* physical way, which is especially helpful if you are struggling to conceive. When you create constructive outlets, they begin to

remember, the goal is to understand one another—not to agree on everything

replace the negative default behaviors you are trying to weed out of your life. And don't forget to take a break from scheduled intimacy now and then, and let yourselves be spontaneous lovers. This is important. Planning a weekend getaway that pulls you out of your ordinary routine and environment can be just the thing that gets you out of a relationship rut.

All of these measures are extremely valuable to help dismantle that barrier blocking your forward momentum in life, but they are not necessarily easy to implement. Pulling yourself out of the confines of treatment may take a concerted effort. There may well be times when you don't *feel* like going anywhere or doing anything different. Feeling this way is okay and very normal. But if you make an effort to do enriching, relationship-building things *anyway,* you will garner great dividends for yourself and your marriage. You will learn that no matter what is happening in your life, you need to make a conscious effort *to grow your relationship.* And, you will discover that it is only in so doing, that your relationship becomes a firm foundation, as well as a soft place to land.

The Case Studies in this Book

Throughout the book, you will find actual case studies from Marina's client files, with the names and identifying personal details changed to protect the individuals involved. These private struggles and breakthroughs illustrate important points made within each chapter. Sometimes what you cannot see in yourself, you will be able to identify in someone else.

In Chapters 3 through 9, (the power tools chapters) you will clearly be able to see and understand the difference the power tools can make in your life. For now, this first case study, which is about Caroline and Steven, will help you to see not only the impact infertility can have on a couple's life, but also see how their baggage affected both their relationship and their struggle.

FROM MARINA'S CASE FILES ON
Caroline and Steven R.

*t*his couple suffers with unexplained infertility. Caroline underwent several trials of IVF. None of these efforts resulted in a pregnancy.

Caroline is the product of divorce and alcoholism and is the oldest of three children. When she was ten years old, her alcoholic father deserted the family. As the oldest child, she was often surrogate mother to her younger siblings, especially while her mother waited tables on the late shift. When her mother returned home from working double shifts, she was usually exhausted and emotionally unavailable. From as far back as Caroline could remember, she was a caregiver. Taking on more than her share of responsibility was always second nature to her, and she learned to go it alone, and never ask for or expect help or support.

In her twenties, she married a man a few years older than she is. At the time, he too was alcoholic, which covered up the fact that he is extremely introverted and not emotionally available. Over the years, the husband stopped drinking, but due to lack of treatment, he still deals with his emotions by withdrawing and disconnecting emotionally. Although their relationship is not marred by any of the turbulence and upheaval that Caroline grew up with, she believes that her relationship with her husband lacks depth, and still feels like she is "going it alone." She longs for a child to fill the empty void within her life.

The couple enters fertility treatment with little communication, as is the norm in their relationship. In fact, the decision to begin treatment is made one day when the couple agrees to babysit for a friend's rambunctious little puppy. The couple, not being dog owners, was unfamiliar with the antics of a little dog. In the midst of the commotion the puppy made, Steven exclaimed, "With all this confusion, we may as well have a child!" Caroline took this as the green light to start treatment.

In typical fashion, Caroline handled the entire treatment process, appointments, procedures, and injections, on her own. Feeling the guilt of being unable to conceive a child, she imagines that this is her due, and it never even occurs to her she can reach out and ask for support. In this, and in countless other ways, Caroline enables Steven to remain dependent in the relationship, treating him more like a younger sibling than her partner. He is the first to say that having a child is mostly "her thing," but he imagines he will adjust once the baby comes.

But a baby doesn't come, and Caroline's deep desire to parent a child takes her to the avenue of adoption. Again, Steven says little, simply going along with the protocol, and involving himself in his own pursuits—mostly, taking tennis lessons, and playing every chance he gets. During the home study, Steven finally discloses his discomfort with taking in a child that is biologically unrelated to him, shattering Caroline's hopes to adopt.

The couple's involvement in counseling allowed them to address the damage wrought by their codependency and poor communication skills. In addition, Steven was able to confront the unfinished business of his alcoholism, and today he continues his recovery work. Both realized the importance of being a team and having balance in their relationship; Caroline realized she needed to let go, while Steven had to learn the skills necessary to step up and take his share of responsibility for the relationship. As both practice their newly acquired communication skills, and what it means for them to be in partnership, they have made the choice to live childfree. Caroline has grieved this loss, but has decided that, since Steven is immovable on this issue, she would rather remain in the marriage.

Today Caroline is knee-deep in volunteer work for her local chapter of Big Brothers/Big Sisters, while partnering with Steven as proud parents of their two Australian shepherds.

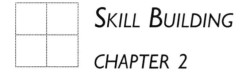

SKILL BUILDING

CHAPTER 2

1. Think back to a time when you felt stressed in some way. What are some of your default behaviors? Does your spouse or partner have default behaviors that you can identify?

2. Pick a time when you and your husband or partner handled a disagreement poorly. Did any of your default behaviors show up there?

3. Pick a time when you handled a conflict well. What did you do differently?

4. What were some things that you and your husband loved to do together when you first got married, but have stopped doing?

5. Is there anything new that you've thought about lately that you think would be great fun to do together?

6. Are you willing to talk to your husband about the two of you revisiting old interests or trying new ones?

7. The baggage that Caroline and Steven brought into their relationship further complicated their struggle with infertility. After you have identified some of your own default behaviors, see if you can also identify how these responses have become ingrained in you. Are you repeating response patterns you saw in your parents? Are you repeating patterns you set up in a previous relationship?

Your First Power Tool: Take Care of Your Body

Take care of your body.
These words sound like such simple advice that it is easy to disregard their real strength. Perhaps your first reaction is to say, "Hey, I already eat right and take my vitamins—what more can I do?" However, taking care of your body while also experiencing the stress of trying to conceive can be different from taking care of your body under other circumstances. Your objectives are different and so are your needs. In many regards, taking care of your body at this time is as much about doing *less* of some things as it is about doing *more* of others.

People often respond positively when given technical-sounding solutions to problems. They don't necessarily put these complex answers to work in their lives, but they tend to feel that something that sounds scientifically advanced has recognizable credibility. In contrast, they frequently brush aside simple answers to problems, perceiving them to be too easy to be effective. Weight loss strategies illustrate a perfect example of this type of erroneous reasoning. Consumers spend millions of dollars each year on

⊞ *your first power tool is: take care of your body*

drugs, herbal wraps, hypnosis, and a laundry list of solutions that promise to help them slim down. While some of these remedies do result in pounds lost, the most effective solution for lasting weight loss is simple: eat less and exercise more.

Many of the solutions for nurturing yourself also sound simplistic. Some may seem so simple that you think they could not possibly produce appreciable results. *Don't buy into that rationale.* With everything that is going on in your life, simple solutions are not merely as good as complicated ones; they are better.

Using your first power tool and taking care of your body is the most fundamental and powerful of all the strategies you have available to help you deal with the challenges of fertility. Taking care of your body is also the power tool over which you personally have the greatest control. Ironically, it can be the most difficult tool to implement because of how you may be experiencing yourself emotionally.

Your fertility struggles may have left you with feelings of anger directed at your body, perhaps even the sense that your body is betraying you. These kinds of feelings make caring for yourself a real challenge. Take a moment to think about this: would you be angry with another woman just because she was struggling to conceive a child?

Of course you wouldn't! In fact, you would be nurturing and supportive. You would recognize that adding to someone else's troubles by mistreating her would only make things worse for that person, and would leave you feeling awful.

The same logic applies to how you treat yourself. Right now, you are that woman, struggling to conceive a child. *Your body* needs you. While it may appear to be uncooperative, in fact, that body of yours is doing its very best. You wouldn't be harsh and angry with someone else in this situation. *So why mistreat yourself?*

You will experience genuine transformation—mentally, physically, and spiritually—if you learn to nurture your body and truly understand that right now, your body is doing the best it can. You and your body are in a lifelong partnership. As much as you think this period in your life is all about what you need from your body, it is much more about *what your body needs from you.* You are in a critical time in your life and it will never be more important than it is right now for you to nurture *you.*

Love Yourself First

If you find that loving yourself is a struggle, try to imagine instead that you are mothering your own body in the same way you hope someday to mother your child. During this time, when there is no baby to pamper, turn your abundance of nurturing feelings inward and focus them on yourself. Giving love to yourself is neither self-centered, nor inappropriate. Instead, loving yourself is the essential first step in genuinely loving others. Your relationships with others are an extension of your relationship with yourself. In making the choice to nurture and care for yourself, you are moving toward being a happier, healthier individual. You will become a better partner for your spouse, and if you do have a child in your life, a better mother to that child. And the first step to doing this is as simple as taking a deep breath.

Breathe In…Breathe Out

Take a deep breath. *No,* take a really deep breath—very slowly. Most people take breathing for granted. They don't think about when or how they do it, and they certainly don't consider that there are right and wrong ways to breathe. But if you are tempted to skip these next pages because you think that you already know everything you need to know about something as fundamental as breathing, *think again.*

Effective breathing is simple, powerful, and free. Doing it properly increases your energy level, stabilizes your mood, decreases anxiety, improves mental focus and concentration, and does a host of wonderful things that enhance the physiological functions of your body. Despite the importance of breathing, most people never master the basic process of exchanging "bad air" for "good air" in the correct and beneficial way. Quite simply, for something a person does an average of 20,000 times a day, many people are doing it incorrectly.

Think about what you did the last time the dentist came toward you with a buzzing, whining dental drill in hand, or how you react when you are startled, or you see an accident that is about to happen.

> *whatever you resist, persists; the more you try to disconnect from the physical part of yourself to avoid painful feelings, the more these feelings will continue*

Most people respond to such stresses by gasping—taking a short, sucking breath of air, or they hold their breath entirely. When circumstances around you feel threatening, your breathing adapts to the classic fight or flight pattern.

Fight or flight breathing routes oxygenated blood to the extremities, preparing your muscles to do battle with the foe or challenge you face. Yet most people don't throw a punch at the dentist, even if their instincts say that he or she is a "threat". The battles you face in your life today are likely to be either verbal conflicts or non-verbalized conflicts that you internalize—not fist fights. Nevertheless, your body reacts to such threats like the real thing. As Gay and Kathryn Hendricks of the Hendricks Institute in California explain in their book, *At the Speed of Life,* "When a person is under a threat, the breathing moves rapidly in the chest, accompanied by massive secretions from the adrenal glands. The heart rate goes up, and the muscles tighten."

You live in a world where wild animals and opposing tribesmen no longer jeopardize your existence. Instead, job loss, family conflict, and an ever-growing stack of bills to pay have replaced such dangers. In addition, thanks to the global outreach of modern news reporting, you experience your own threats and dangers along with the hurricanes, typhoons, mudslides, wild fires, avalanches, famine, floods, and acts of terrorism and warfare confronting every other person on the planet. You react by perceiving a threat, whether or not there directly is one. The effect that real or perceived threats have on the body is what is commonly known as "stress."

Stress causes significant and dramatic bodily changes, but unless you actually double up your fists and physically fight, or you take flight by running from the danger as far and as fast as you can, your body has no way to dispel the physiological overload it is experiencing. Instead, you stand in the moment, taking shallow breaths, rerouting your oxygenated blood supply away from your brain. Because saber-tooth tigers or marauding pillagers no longer challenge your daily survival, annoyances like traffic jams, an irritable boss, or a moment of conflict with your spouse or co-worker will trigger your fight or flight reaction.

Okay, now exhale.

You can change your breathing patterns. You can replace a habit that does not serve you well with a new pattern that not only prevents unnecessary bodily stress reactions, but also reduces the impact of other unavoidable stress triggers. *You can breathe like a baby.*

Watch sleeping babies or toddlers and you will see that in their natural breathing pattern—relaxed or asleep—their bellies rise and fall with each breath. Once upon a time, you were that baby. Your breathing was natural, rhythmic, and sufficiently deep that you filled the lower part of your lungs with oxygen. Your belly rose and fell gently with each peaceful breath. Then life happened, and the everyday stress you experienced became locked inside your body. You responded by taking shallow breaths.

If you are like most people, each day you experience more things that create stress than things that relieve stress. Over time, the imbalance between stress makers and stress relievers causes you routinely to breathe from the upper part of your lungs without properly involving the lower parts. In short, you turn your breathing from right side up, to upside down.

To get a better understanding of how this happens, take a moment and try a simple experiment. Close your eyes and place one hand on your chest and the other on your belly. Think of an everyday stressful occurrence. Make it something simple, like being stuck in traffic and knowing that you are going to be late for an important appointment. Breathe for a minute and observe what is happening. Which of your hands rises and falls more, the one on your chest or the one on your belly? Is your breathing slow and deep, or is it shallow?

Now, close your eyes again. This time, think about a **time in your life that was stress-free and relaxing, perhaps a day at the beach, or having lunch with a close friend.** Let your breathing occur naturally, again placing one hand lightly on your belly and one hand lightly on your chest. Note which hand moves more, and whether your breathing slows down or speeds up.

What do these two exercises tell you? In the first experiment, it is a good guess that the hand on your chest moved more than did the hand resting on your belly. It's probably also true that you felt your muscles get tense and your breathing become short and shallow as you imagined a stressful situation. What you observed was your fight or flight response kicking into gear. Even though there was no real danger, your body still reacted as if the threat was real. The fact that you conjured up this feeling in your imagination indicates that even *thinking* stressful thoughts produces stress-based body responses.

Even more important than the first exercise is the insight you gain from the second one. If you are like most people, when you tried breathing the second time, **in a more relaxed state,** the hand on your chest still moved more than did the hand on your belly. Your body remained locked in upside down breathing—the shorter, more shallow breaths associated with stress response. Over time, shallow breathing is exhausting to the body and may lead to the types of stress-related ailments everyone is so familiar with today. The emotional toll can also be high. The chronic release of stress-related hormones can result in hormone overload followed by hormone depletion. Simply correcting faulty breathing patterns can, and will, be an enormous help in relieving many long-term, low-grade feelings of confusion, fatigue, anxiety, and depression.

Your first step in taking care of your body and creating a personal breakthrough in the midst of the life crisis of infertility is to help your body relearn proper breathing. In order to do this, you need to understand what happens to your body when you breathe optimally. Each time you inhale with a full deep breath, the diaphragm, behind the sternum, moves down into the belly, expanding it a bit and making more space for the lungs to fill with air. When you exhale, the lungs contract with the release of air and the diaphragm returns to its place behind the sternum. The belly relaxes.

To see this in action, take a closer look at the baby mentioned earlier.

Watch how a baby breathes, say after nursing or when at rest. You will notice that it is as if her entire body breathes. With every inhale, her belly swells effortlessly, as the pelvis rocks up a bit. Then, with every exhale, her belly relaxes, and the small of her back flattens. This cycle illustrates the body breathing optimally.

Unfortunately, over time, improper breathing causes the diaphragm muscle to lose tone. Out of condition, the diaphragm no longer facilitates proper breathing. Yet like any other muscle in your body, the right exercises will tone and condition your diaphragm. The following simple core breathing exercise is an ideal way to recondition the diaphragm, so that it becomes more responsive to proper breathing during the day. This exercise helps you correct and relearn proper breathing.

Core Breathing Exercise

Lie on a mat on the floor. Bend your knees and place your feet about hip-width apart. Inhale slowly to a count of four, allowing your belly to swell, and your pelvis to rock up naturally. Stop for a count of one at the top of the breath, and then slowly exhale, to a count of four, allowing the belly to relax and the back to flatten. Start with a minute of breathing, about six full in-out breathing cycles, slowly increasing to five minutes, as you become more comfortable.

It is perfectly normal if this exercise feels a little choppy at first. Placing your hand or a book on your stomach may help you ensure that primarily your belly, rather than your chest, is rising and falling. Try to breathe through your nose, because your nose has fine hairs that serve as a filtering system for unwanted bacteria or inhaled irritants. You may also find that you feel a little dizzy when you first start these exercises. If that happens, don't worry—your body may not be used to taking in so much oxygen! Just go slowly, and be consistent. Before long, you'll find that your breathing feels full and easy. This exercise is an ideal way to begin and end your day.

Core breathing is a wonderful way to kick the stress habit and refocus on your body during the day. One excellent suggestion, when you are re-training your breathing, is to leave yourself little sticky notes to remind you to take a core breath now and then. Place them on your bathroom mirror, the dashboard of your car; even use the message as your screen saver at work. Then, any time you are feeling particularly stressed, you can instantly decompress by taking the core breathing exercise and making it vertical—simply doing it when you are in an upright position. No matter where you are, take a long, slow, deep breath to a count of four. Breathe deeply into your lungs, letting your ribs and belly expand a bit. Hold for one count, and then slowly exhale to a count of four, allowing your belly to relax into your spine. Repeat four times.

You may need a little self-reminding to get on the right breathing track, but the rewards are well worth it. More energy, increased ability to focus and concentrate, and a greater feeling of overall wellbeing is commonplace. Relearning correct breathing is simple, easy to implement, and free. You have nothing to lose (except unwanted stress and stress symptoms) by try-ing it, and everything to gain. Proper breathing is the foundation of any solid self-care program and it is a critical step in putting your first power tool to work in caring for your body.

Breathing Your Way to Wholeness

Proper breathing is not only a master key to physiological wellbeing; it is an essential element in emotional wholeness as well. As simplistic as it may sound, as you breathe more fully, you open the door to the possibility of experiencing life more fully.

Does this sound strange?

Think of your body as a container, and your breathing as an opening that determines whether, and to what extent, emotional experiences may enter. Breathe fully, and you feel fully; breathe shallowly, and your emotional experience diminishes.

To illustrate this more clearly, go back to the exercise in which you assessed your breathing while imagining a stressful event. Even though this event existed only in your imagination, your body responded to it as if it were real. Your stress response triggered breathing that was short and tense. In essence, you tried to resist the unpleasant memory of your emotional experience by tensing your muscles and breathing shallowly. This is the same way your body attempts to block emotional experience.

"So what?" you may be thinking. "If I breathe in a way that minimizes unpleasant feelings, isn't that a good thing?"

Unfortunately, the answer to that question is an unequivocal "no!" The truth is, *whatever you resist, persists*. This means that the more you try to disconnect from the physical part of yourself to avoid painful feelings, the more these feelings continue to exist. At the time unpleasant emotions crop up, you may believe that you are able to sidestep the feelings you want to avoid. But feelings do not go away because you decide to ignore them. Emotions are energy and as Einstein and the laws of thermodynamics tell us, "…energy cannot be destroyed."

Your feelings never really go away. Unless you acknowledge them for what they are, they simply go underground either to fester, or to boil over like water heated too long, too hot in a teakettle. Anytime you find yourself overreacting about something insignificant, you are demonstrating how built up emotional energy will discharge itself any way it can.

Getting stuck in an unhealthy breathing pattern causes you to resist not only unpleasant emotional experiences, but *all* of your emotional experiences—positive as well as negative. Your feelings of joy, sexuality, enthusiasm, and overall wellbeing, are all diminished—*compromised.* You feel less powerful, less connected, and less in your body than you should be able to feel.

Core breathing provides a wonderful solution. Breathing fully into your feelings—*all of them*—is the antidote to restricting your breathing in an effort to insulate yourself from your feelings. Breathing into your feelings is *the* way to connect with them, and by so doing, make more conscious, resourceful choices.

Now for some women, the idea of breathing into and fully experiencing unpleasant feelings may feel like a daunting task. Conditioning tells you to divide feelings into two categories: good or bad. For example, most people would say that happiness and joy are *good* feelings and anger and fear are *bad* feelings. But, in reality, feelings are neither good nor bad; they just are. You may enjoy experiencing some feelings more than you enjoy experiencing others. The feelings themselves, however, are not the bad guys; they are simply emotional reactions based on your perceptions of life's events. Acknowledging your feelings for what they are allows you to realize that you are in charge and that you get to decide whether to express the energy from these emotions in positive ways, rather than negative ones.

Allowing yourself to consciously experience and embody a full range of feelings is the essence of being fully human. Take long, slow, centered breaths into *all* of your feelings. You will be permitting each feeling to expand, express, and then to process through. Clients often remark that breathing into their feelings allows them to experience their emotions like the action of a wave; after a momentary expansion, the feeling simply washes through. Breathing fully is an excellent way to step into your feelings and to embrace the wholeness of your experiences.

Breathing fully through feelings is also a way to transform an emotion. As noted psychologist and the founder of Gestalt Therapy, Fritz Pearls explains, "fear is excitement without the breath." Breathing through your feelings allows even an emotion like fear to transform itself into one of exhilaration and excitement. In this way, it is possible to become a master of your own experiences. Rather than wasting energy to stay vigilant and avoid feelings that you anticipate will be unpleasant, you can efficiently use your energy to *breathe* into your experiences, transform them, and to feel fully alive.

That Healing Touch

When you were a child and you hurt your knee, you probably went straight to your mother for comfort. Much of the time, you needed only a hug, a kiss, and perhaps a small bandage added for effect. Miraculously when you received this nurturing attention, you felt better—the hurt just seemed to go away.

A mother's comfort heals hurts in part because the loving attention distracts the injured child, and also because it brings the child back to a familiar place within herself, where she previously experienced and savored being the focus of her mother's caregiving. The presence of a parent's tenderness also causes the child to relax muscles that have tensed with anxiety or pain. When the muscles relax, blood flow returns to normalcy throughout the body, breathing patterns improve, and miraculously, the pain of the child's injury actually does subside. When your body undergoes stress, you too, need comfort and nurturing to alleviate the tension and to help you relax. Massage provides a perfect answer.

Massage is an excellent way to care for your b
relieve those worldly tensions that seem to settle
become trapped inside of you. Massage has existed
and probably evolved from the natural instinct to "
whenever one is hurting. As far back as 3000 B.C., the ..cluded
massage in their prescription for complete health, and m..ssage therapy is
documented in the ancient civilizations of the Greeks and Hindus as well.

The massage system of kneading and stroking not only feels wonderful, it stimulates, relaxes, and tones the body. The benefits reach deep into
layers of muscle, increasing flexibility, stimulating the circulation, and sup-
porting the lymphatic system. In addition, massage releases endorphins,
the body's natural painkiller, making massage an ideal way to control and
alleviate pain, and deal with chronic, physical conditions.

The physical benefits are only part of the story, however. In 1986.
Touch Research Institute at the University of Miami conducted gr
breaking research. The research, conducted on premature babies
fect example of the invisible seam that connects body and soul

The preterm babies were divided into two groups. The
tween the two groups were consistent, with one differenc
received massage therapy. The results were astonishing–
who received massage therapy showed forty-seven
gain, and a six-day shorter hospital stay, than di
not receiving massage!

Fortunately, such profound benefits are
ing of being touched in a safe, compass
ence—one that heals the body and calr
the demands and expectations you are
extremely important that you make time to

y to make regular massages a part of your life, and as you do, be particularly mindful of one thing: *be with* your experience. This means, rather
than allowing yourself to be distracted or to talk with your massage therapist, make this time only about you. Listen to your body and keep coming
back to yourself, bringing your attention to where the therapist's hands are
working. Breathe into any tension or tightness. A lot of stress is stored in
the body, so breathing into all those little spaces that you normally ignore,
allows you to unwind and meet that emotional tension where it's housed.
The results—a relaxed body and a restored spirit—are well worth it.

You Are What You Eat and Drink or Fail to Eat or Drink

Many people today are fortunate to live in a land of abundance, where
food and drink are as accessible as their refrigerator or the neighborhood
grocery store. Yet the adage, "you are what you eat," is probably never more
true than when you are hoping for a child. Paying attention to your diet is
essential so that you know you are doing all you can to create an optimal
conception environment. In terms of *quality*, it is important to understand
eating (and drinking) for two starts before pregnancy.

Water covers approximately seventy-five percent of the earth's surface—
exactly the same percentage of water within the human body. This
ing parallel between you and Mother Earth is further extended by
that both systems are fragilely dependant on maintaining their wa-
e. Most people already understand that their body can live days,
without food, but can only survive a very short time without
rch sources differ, as do the needs of one individual to another,
re between seventy-five and eighty-five percent of the brain is
ween eighty and ninety-five percent of the blood is water.

Even though water is the most abundant substance both on earth and in our bodies, most
people walk around suffering—by choice—from
some degree of dehydration. Unrecognized dehy-

⊞ *garbage in;*
garbage out

dration occurs because there is a tendency to use thirst as a barometer of
how much to drink. Unfortunately, by the time you feel thirsty, your body
is already advancing beyond the early stages of dehydration.

Replenishing the eighty or more ounces (approximately 2.5 liters) of
water your body loses each day is critical. Doing so ensures that all of your
body systems function at their best possible level. Putting back as much
fluid as you are naturally losing sustains your clarity of thought and helps
your body maintain its critical chemical balance.

Like proper breathing, this first piece of nutritional advice is simple,
free, and readily accessible. Make it a point to drink plenty of water each
day. Make it convenient—keep an insulated water bottle with you, so that
it is always within easy reach. Try using a straw, which seems naturally to
increase the amount you tend to drink, or adding a splash of fruit juice or
a squeeze of fresh lemon or lime for variety.

Choose water over other beverages as often as you can, especially in fa-
vor of beverages that contain caffeine. Numerous studies have linked caffeine, found in coffee, teas, colas, and chocolate, to both reduced fertility
and to increased risk of miscarriage. Cutting back or entirely eliminating
caffeine consumption is an excellent idea.

The advice that works so well for caffeine is even more critical when
it comes to alcohol. Alcohol's adverse effect on the fetus, and the need to
give it up completely while pregnant, are well documented. However, the
truth is, alcohol's impact on *fertility* has not been well studied. Although
having a glass of wine on occasion is unlikely to be a problem, many

experts recommend that, since alcohol can affect hormone levels, it is best to play it safe and forego alcohol completely, as soon as you begin trying to conceive.

While the message may be pretty clear-cut about what to drink, when it comes to what to eat, there is a lot of conflicting information. The easiest way to cut through all the confusing, and often times contradictory information is to remember that *you are a biochemical being.* How you fuel yourself and how you run your engine is paramount to how your machine functions. The adage, "garbage in, garbage out," certainly applies here. If you want your vehicle to function at its best, feed it with the highest quality fuel you can. Eat healthful nourishing meals and snacks of high quality protein and complex carbohydrates. Savor the look and taste of deeply colored fruits and vegetables and dense and textured whole grains. Make sure you do not go long periods without food, because this causes your blood sugar to plummet and fosters irritability, moodiness, anxiety, depression, and hormonal imbalance. Avoid diets that reduce caloric intake to the point that your metabolism slows, as this not only contributes to weight gain, it may also predispose you to depression. Look for sources of slow burning, consistent fuel in order to stabilize both your moods and your energy levels.

In addition, when your goal is to become pregnant, it is important that you keep your weight within a normal range. Studies have shown that because of the hormonal implications, women who are either too thin or too heavy, have a more difficult time conceiving and responding to fertility medication, a fact that authors Alice Domar and Alice Lesch address in their book, *Conquering Infertility: Dr. Alice Domar's Mind/Body Guide to Enhancing Fertility and Coping with Infertility.* An easy way to calculate your ideal weight is to look at your body-mass index, or BMI. In order to determine your BMI, multiply your weight in pounds by 703, and then divide that amount by your height in inches, squared.

A BMI between 20 and 25 is optimum in terms of fertility, so you may want to gain or lose a few pounds. If you need to make a dramatic change in your weight, or if eating well is new to you, don't attempt to go it alone. Seeking the advice of a qualified dietician can be an enormous asset in retraining your eating habits, as well as providing you the tools you need to create a healthful diet for the family you are creating. Be sure that you also discuss vitamins and mineral supplements with your healthcare provider. For example, it is a good idea to take a one-a-day type multi-vitamin, or a pre-natal vitamin that contains folic acid, as this has been found to be specifically important, during not only pregnancy but also prior to conception. On the other hand, an over-consumption of other vitamins, including A and D, has been linked to birth defects. In addition, be aware of any herbal supplements you are taking or are considering because some herbs can impact medications, or even contain impurities, such as lead. Thoroughly discuss with your physician, anything you take by prescription or over the counter.

Food and Mood

Amazingly, just making different choices in the things you take into your body can make significant difference in your health and emotional wellbeing. The evidence that backs this up is indisputable. One study in particular (the 2002 London-based *Food and Mood* project) found that almost ninety percent of participants increased their energy and improved their emotional states by simply reducing their intake of "stressors" such as sugar, caffeine, alcohol, and chocolate, and increasing their consumption of supporters such as vegetables, fruit, and water. This is powerful information, especially at a time in your life when the stress of infertility can compromise both your physical wellbeing and your emotional state.

Knowledge is power, so choose wisely! On special occasions, let yourself indulge in your grandmother's pumpkin pie, that piece of wedding cake, or your mother-in-law's yummy cannoli. For your day-to-day healthful diet, focus on the fresh, healthy, natural foods your body requires.

On a final note, perhaps no discussion about food would be complete without considering the emotional relationships so intertwined with food and all things associated with eating. Many wonderful memories and life events, as well as satisfying moments, are built around the simple pleasure of good food. The sharing of food is an integral aspect of solid family life and cultural heritages. Food is an important part of holidays and celebrations, and the preparation of a simple meal can be a welcome respite at the end of a busy day. Certainly, you do not want to stop enjoying food, or deprive yourself of its feel, taste, delightful aromas, and beautiful presentations. Nevertheless, when food becomes comfort, reward, or the enemy—well, that's a problem, and that attitude is sure to contaminate any positive choices you attempt to make.

Stressful emotions are part of life, but if you are struggling to conceive, you are sure to experience more than your share of them. In a moment of weakness, you may be tempted to think that food can provide a quick and easy solace to your woes. If you have ever felt this way, you are not alone. In one study documented in the *Journal of Applied Social Psychology* (1996) and featured in a 2004 *CBS News Healthwatch*[4] segment entitled, "Stressed Women Seek Fatty Food," highly frustrated women ate twice the amount of fatty foods that unstressed women ate. And as everyone who has been there knows, this is a trap, and the momentary gratification you may feel

---

[4] See website: http://www.cbsnews.com/stories/2004/07/06/health/main627835.shtml

by indulging in some unhealthy food choice, only ends up causing you more stress in the long run.

in one study... highly stressed women ate twice the amount of fatty food that unstressed women ate

The solution is two-fold. First, it is important to understand that only when you stop giving food power that it was never meant to have, will you see it as the wonderful sustenance it was meant to be. Secondly, it is critical that you proactively incorporate into your life effective ways to really bust through stress: breathe properly, drink water, eat well, and of course, get moving!

Get Moving

Do you recall being four years old, or eight, or ten, and standing in the middle of a room twirling and spinning? Do you remember running as hard and as fast as you could so you wouldn't be tagged as "it" in the recess game of chase? Or being fourteen and dancing in front of the mirror that hung on the back of your bedroom door?

As a child, you moved with glee and abandon. You did it because it was fun. If you spun in circles until you tumbled to the floor or tried to turn cartwheels but landed on the just-mown summer grass, it was perfectly okay. You were not self-conscious about how you looked when you moved, nor did you need a choreographed plan, or even a reason for twirling, jumping, dancing, or leaping. You had the natural instinct to realize that moving not only felt good when you did it, but left you with a lingering upbeat feeling and exuberance about life and about yourself. In fact, there is a real link between exercise and the power it has to evoke those wonderful feelings of wellbeing. While the link has been proven time and again, one particular study, conducted in 2005 by the University of Texas Southwestern Medical

you and your body are one—an integrated system—which can work in harmony

Center, Alberta Children's Hospital and the Cooper Institute,[5] looked solely at the impact of exercise on depression. The findings revealed that people who exercised thirty minutes for three to five times each week, showed a fifty percent drop in mild to moderate depression. Even people who only exercised moderately registered a thirty percent decline in depressive symptoms. No drugs, no therapy, just exercise. Children, when left to their own devices, often naturally understand what is good for them.

That body of yours, originally designed to fend off unwanted advances from Neanderthal men and attacks by wild animals, was meant to move. When you restrict your physical movement, you create an unhealthy chemical imbalance within your body's systems, much like going through life at full speed yet never shifting out of low gear or never disengaging the parking brake on your car. Damage will occur!

One of the unique challenges when you are trying to conceive comes in finding the correct balance between too little exercise and too much. Even though exercise is essential to your overall health and wellbeing, during the time you are attempting to conceive, you must approach exercise cautiously. Intense exercise can halt the body from ovulating and even menstruating. Listen to your body and do not overdo it. Try walking instead of running, or Pilates or yoga instead of high-intensity aerobics. Look for every opportunity you can to move without using this period of your life to train for a marathon. Take the stairs, park your car on the far side of the parking lot, and stretch regularly while you are at your desk. Keep reinforcing your natural, human instinct to move.

---

[5] See website: http://www.innovations-report.com/html/reports/medicine_health/report-39334.html

Loving Yourself Into Wholeness

How you perceive yourself, and the choices you make, has everything to do with whether you have a loving relationship with your body. If you ask most people where inside their bodies they live, they will identify that they live in their chests because that is where their heart is, or that they live in their heads, because that is where the brain is housed. But what if you were able to achieve the feeling that you live inside all of your body? What if you could feel as if the part of you that is "you" was not merely housed in some sectioned-off corner of your physical body, but actually embodied every inch of you—from your fingertips to your toes to your ears and even your elbows? What would it be like to live in, and love, the whole of yourself?

When you lose sight of this innate and intimate relationship, it becomes easy to disconnect from your body, and stop moving. The less you move, the more the disconnect increases. Modern lifestyles have made it easy to go through your day moving as little as possible in order to accomplish your routine tasks. You let the electric can opener open the can of coffee in the morning, turn on the little robot vacuum cleaner to clean the bedroom carpet, drive to work in a car with "power everything," and then take the elevator upstairs to your office. There, you sit in your ergonomic chair and move as little as possible throughout your day. You lose that subtle feeling of satisfaction that comes from using your body to do even little things. A chasm develops between your mind and your body, and when you do think about your body, you snort in disgust because it does not look like you want it to look. Compound this with fertility struggles, and the chasm grows wider as you judge your body for not responding the way you want it to respond. Your body feels foreign, as if it exists separately and apart from you.

Get up. Stand in the middle of the floor and twirl around in circles.

Leap, sway, or pirouette—just move. Move your body until the joy you felt as a child begins to filter back into your spirit. You do not have to look good doing it. You are not training for the Olympics or trying to win a body building title. You are moving because failure to move is unhealthy for your body *and* for your mind. You are moving because it is natural to move. Release the part of you that is "you" from the tiny corner it now occupies inside your body, and in so doing, let your mind and your body reconnect as they were meant to—as a single functioning unit. Your body cannot betray you if you recognize that you and your body are not separate units working independently from each other. You and your body are one—an integrated system, which can work in harmony. Each part functions best when you love, nurture, and recognize both parts as the powerful contributors to your total wellbeing that they really are.

The Power Tool to Keep You Going and Going and Going

While writing this chapter, Marina wrote in her original notes, "The entire premise of Chapter 3 is to let the reader know she can transcend the crappy feelings she has about her body not doing what she wants. She can replace them with caring feelings and actions. She can learn to actually use this experience with infertility as an opportunity to heal her relationship with her body." The two authors did not intend for the note, typed in an e-mail exchange, ever to make it to the final draft. But pages and pages could be written that do not sum up the first tool for how to turn your life crisis into a powerful, personal breakthrough as clearly as do these few sentences. Use your experience of infertility to transcend a negative approach and replace it with a positive approach.

Your first power tool is, "take care of your body." Your body is not a shell you inhabit or vessel in which your spirit dwells. Your body and your psyche are inseparably intertwined and they must function as one unit. Whatever you do to one, you do just as much to the other. Rather than feeling frustration over what your body is or is not doing, choose to remind yourself daily that your body is doing the very best it

rather than feeling frustration over what your body is or is not doing, you can remind yourself daily that your body is doing the very best it can

can. Replace your feelings of frustration with feelings of self-care and self-nurturing. If you do not love yourself *yet*, that's okay. Start by being *willing* to take this step, to being open to this invitation. There is an enormous amount of power in simply declaring your intention to move toward this goal. Unless you open this door, there is little chance that you can properly execute the first power tool and take care of your body.

Taking care of your body, in all the ways suggested here, might increase your odds of conceiving a child. More importantly, taking care of your body *will* improve your physical and mental health, and will make it easier for you to live a quality life during this period that could otherwise be overshadowed by all that accompanies infertility and its challenges.

FROM MARINA'S CASE FILES ON
Sabre and Jonas K.

*t*he first time Sabre shuffled into my office, her posture told the whole story. Slumped over, eyes downcast, Sabre looked more like a war refugee than the attractive, thirty-seven year old woman she was. As I soon found out, my first impression was accurate—Sabre was barely surviving her own fertility battles.

Sabre's husband initiated her entry into treatment. She related that he was convinced that if only she could become successful in having a child, the depression with which she suffered would "miraculously" lift. Sabre stated she had suffered from low-grade depression for the past five years, almost the length of time she had been undergoing infertility treatment. Her symptoms included frequent tears, anxiety, difficulty focusing and making decisions, irritability, and disrupted sleep. She stated that she had "bad days" once or twice a week, and as a result was only able to work sporadically as a substitute teacher.

Although in fertility treatment for the last five years, Sabre's fertility issues actually stemmed from childhood. A series of surgeries for a congenital defect, treated at age four, left Sabre with only one ovary, and adhesions so severe that natural fertilization was impossible. After several attempts at IVF, testing determined that not only were her eggs not viable, but that she would be unable to carry a child as well. Needless to say, this was a tremendous loss for the couple, especially for Sabre. But rather than grieve, she dutifully followed her husband's lead as he doggedly scheduled appointment after appointment with leading specialists, to not only confirm the accuracy of the initial diagnosis, but also take them to what eventually became the recommended course of treatment: gestational carrier with an egg donor.

"I feel like a shadow of myself," Sabre related during session, "almost like an outside observer in my own life." By the time I saw Sabre in treatment, the couple had already exhausted the services of two gestational carriers, both unable to become pregnant. The donors, two so far, had been each of Sabre's two sisters. "I want to be done," Sabre says, almost to herself. "I want to get on with my life."

Jonas agreed that he would be willing to accompany Sabre into counseling. When he came to my office, what I encountered was a man who deeply longed for a child, and felt helpless to alleviate his wife's suffering. Jonas was on his second marriage, and his first wife was also unable to have a child. Well into his forties, he felt desperate— like he was running out of time. He wanted a child and he wanted his wife to care for this child. He was convinced that once his wife had a baby, she would bond and they would be a family.

Fortunately, during the course of couples counseling, Jonas was able to become aware of the depths of his wife's despair and agreed to put a temporary hold on continued fertility treatment. With the pressure of a baby eased for now, Sabre started to explore her own issues, and how she had used her depression to mask her grief and shut down her feelings. She began to acknowledge the enormous shame she had felt at being unable to conceive and carry a child, as well as the deep sadness at disappointing her husband. Ironically, although these feelings compelled her to follow her husband's lead in fertility treatment, she realized she was angry at him for being so driven for a child. At times, she felt he barely seemed to notice her. Rather than communicating this directly, Sabre used her depression not only to shut down her feelings, but also to act them out. She knew he hated it when she withdrew, and the depression allowed her to do that. This got his attention and allowed her to communicate her hostility.

Once Sabre realized she was already communicating—but in nonverbal and destructive ways—things began to turn around. As she gave herself time to grieve her own loss, and identify and put language to her own feelings, real communication began. Sabre also realized that her deep shame caused her to abandon herself. She needed to learn skills to heal and to care for herself once again. As she realized that her body was not "betraying" her, but in fact, simply doing the best it could, she was able to treat it compassionately. This caused a shift in her self-care, and she began to eat better, to exercise, and to treat her body as a gift.

Over time, her depression lifted. Fortunately, Jonas proved eager to reconnect with his wife, finally admitting that he felt desperate to reach her, and he had believed that having a child was the only way. He too, became aware of the depth of his own grief, and the loss of the child he had hoped to create with his wife. As the couple learned to talk to one another, they agreed to terminate fertility treatment and give themselves time to explore other ways to be a family.

The couple ended treatment, grateful for the growth they had achieved, and their newfound reconnection to one another. Months later, I was happy to receive an announcement and photo in the mail, celebrating the arrival of Anisa, their beautiful little daughter from China.

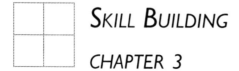

SKILL BUILDING

CHAPTER 3

1. Take an honest self-inventory. Spend a few minutes and write down how you feel about yourself in light of your struggle with fertility. Just listen to your own thoughts and write without thinking, without stopping. When you're done, look at what you've written. Does it reflect a loving, nurturing relationship with yourself, or a critical, judgmental one?

2. How's your breathing? Do the self-check exercise and see whether you tend to breathe through your chest, or in a more centered way. Can you commit to practicing the core breathing exercise for two minutes, morning and evening?

3. How does your relationship with yourself reflect in your lifestyle choices? Do you make food choices to nourish yourself, or do you use food to deal with stress or negative emotions? Are you using physical activity as both an emotional outlet, and for your physical wellbeing? Or are you a couch potato who looks for every opportunity to *not* move?

4. List three things that you are willing to do to get your food and exercise program into gear. Can you call on a friend who will support you in this (a walking buddy, for example), or to whom you can be accountable?

5. Make an appointment for a massage and consider including this in your regular self-care regimen—even if it's only once a month. If cost is a consideration, and you live near a school that teaches massage, you may be able to schedule massages at reduced rates from students in training. Also, look for spas or wellness centers that may offer lower rates when you purchase a series of massages. Supplement this with hand or foot massages—*for and from your partner*. This is a great way to be loving and

nurturing to each other, and to remind yourselves that being intimate doesn't always need to be linked to sex and baby-making.

6. Take a closer look at Sabre and Jonas. Are there ways you act out your feelings that are not productive, and that perhaps even hurt your relationship? If you could put these behaviors into words, what would they be saying?

CHAPTER 4

Your Second Power Tool: Make Conscious Choices

Fertility challenges are a leviathan in your path; fertility challenges are a journey. You read it in the beginning of this book. Nice mental pictures, but can you actually relate them to the confusion and frustration you currently feel?

Most cultures resolve difficult situations by assigning blame and determining retribution—the "penalty" the guilty party must pay. You grew up with this concept as a child, when your parents taught you to own up to what you had done wrong. In elementary school, the teacher would fix her sternest gaze on the classroom of silent students and say, "The person who did this needs to come forward."

Identifying the guilty party, substantiating his or her guilt publicly, and then leveling a penalty on the convicted person is the basis for most judicial systems. Even the language of a religious confessional begins with, "Forgive me Father, for I have sinned...".

If you do not blame yourself for the problem of infertility, who are you

⊞ *your second power tool is: make conscious choices*

going to blame? There has to be someone to blame, right? And it might as well be you.

But what happens when you blame yourself?

You feel guilty.

And what happens when you feel guilty?

You punish yourself.

Yes, that's right, guilt always *draws* punishment. One hundred percent of the time. When you feel guilty enough about something, you find ways to punish yourself, whether you are conscious of doing so or not. So how in the world can you ever get to a place of healing from where you are now?

You have to take "blame" out of the equation, out of your vocabulary, and out of your thought processes. You will never be able to carry out the first power tool of taking care of yourself as long as you feel like you should be punishing your guilty body. Learning to stop affixing blame on yourself will open you up to learning to love and care for your body (Power Tool One) and then to being able to make conscious choices that serve you (Power Tool Two).

In infertility, there is no guilty party to punish, and if there were, your name wouldn't even come up on the list of suspects. You did not cause infertility to happen to you. You are not going through this because you ate or drank the wrong thing. Nor are you experiencing this as punishment for something you did or did not do. Even if your infertility is linked to the age at which you first started trying to conceive, you are still not at fault. You made life decisions based on what seemed best and the information you had at the time.

Get out of the time-out chair you've been sitting in as punishment. Quit laying the blame on yourself, or even worse, laying it on your body as if your physical body is something separate, that stands apart from your mental being. Even prisoners come to the end of their sentence; so if you have been a victim of your own blame game, decide right now that you are done. Declare yourself a free woman.

Allowing misplaced self-blame doesn't bring any closure or sense of justice served when the issue is infertility. Blaming yourself for your situation means only that your emotional growth screeches to a halt and you may very well live the rest of your life with the same anger, guilt, and frustration you are dealing with now. Like Michelle at the beginning of the book, who still felt angry despite giving birth to a biological child, carrying around guilt sets up a situation you never, ever get over.

The truth is, life really *is* a journey. You are only going to be able to make the trip if you first fortify your body with care and nurturing, and then you learn ways to experience and grow through your emotions, rather than shun them.

In order to take off the yoke of guilt, try carrying out your own judicial process. Imagine that you have the task of convincing a jury of twelve that you are the cause of your own fertility struggle. Imagine a jury of your peers: women, some older, some younger, some pregnant, some unable to have children, others who are mothers. Think about the arguments you would present in order to prove your point. Would you win your case? Would you be able to convince even one person on the jury of your guilt?

Of course not! The judge and jury would throw your case out of court for lack of evidence.

When you can accept that there are no good arguments for your own guilt, or the way you've been punishing yourself, you can begin the process of healing. This acceptance will let you take one more important step toward becoming whole and happy, and will leave you feeling as if an enormous weight has been removed from your life. Then, and only then, will you be ready to face the challenges inherent in learning to make conscious *choices*—challenges that can come from the inside as well as the outside.

Women Have Come a Long Way...Or Have They?

Many anthropologists consider the Bushmen who inhabited southern Africa and later the Kalahari Desert, to be descendants of the first inhabitants on earth. Scientists know with certainty that the Bushmen, also called the San, have inhabited that region for at least 20,000 years. They were never an agricultural people; instead, they were the first culture of hunter-gatherers.

The males in the Bushman culture moved through life in a linear fashion. They hunted. They tracked the gemsbok, antelopes, and giraffe of the veldt (open grassland) and when the animals paused, they paused too, waiting for the right moment to strike their prey.

The females in Bushman society were the gatherers. They moved across the arid land, scanning left and right for a withered stem that indicated an edible root buried beneath the hard, dry earth. Occasionally they would be lucky enough to find ostrich eggs or small rodents to add to their simple meals.

As the women searched for food, they watched over the infants and children. They were responsible to make the temporary camps, prepare and cook the food, care for the ill and elderly, create the family's clothing from animal skins, and use found objects to craft all of their own cooking implements, food and water containers, and many of the tools used by their clan.

caretaking can be another word for control

The men? Well, they just hunted. When they finished hunting, they liked to sit by the fire, tell stories of the hunt, and puff on hand rolled smokes.

Sound familiar?

Okay, now fast-forward about 20,000 years, and see how much, or how little, things have changed. If the Bushman's lifestyle doesn't seem familiar, then just think back to the last family gathering or neighborhood cookout you attended. The men might have cooked the steaks on the grill and maybe even played some games with the children, but for the most part, the women in attendance planned the gathering, prepared the food, watched over the children, and when it was all done, cleaned up after the event. So is it any wonder that even now, it feels almost instinctive for women to put their own needs second, while they put the needs of others first? Women have done this for generations and generations, and such age-old patterns are very hard to break.

For the most part, women gear their lives more toward multi-tasking than do men. The fact that Bushmen women, and thousands of generations since, have taken care of everyone else's needs, (often at the expense of their own) could have as much to do with physiology as with sociology. Numerous sources, including *The Female Brain* by Dr. Louann Brizendine, show that there is much more than social conditioning behind the fact that women wind up managing a diversity of responsibilities and doing so in ways that are very different from how men function and act.

The wiring in women's brains is actually different from that in men's brains. Dr. Brizendine is the founder of the Women's Mood and Hormone Clinic in the Department of Psychiatry at the University of California, San Francisco. As she explains, the female brain develops the ability to read facial expressions and inflections in speech at an early age and to a far greater degree than does the male brain. This survival-linked skill may have always been part of the female make-up or may have evolved through selective mutation. Either way, as Brizendine says, "If you can read faces and voices, you can…predict what a bigger, more aggressive male is going to do. And since you're smaller, you probably need to band with other females to fend off attacks from a ticked off caveman." Brizendine describes such attributes as being "hardwired into the brains of women."

As children, girls play together in small groups, often even calling themselves a club. As members of the group or club, they are emotionally connected. When one girl is sad, the other girls openly comfort her sadness and share in her unhappiness. When one girl is injured or ill, play stops for everyone. The group tends to her needs, worries about the situation, and collectively mothers her. This common scenario happens across cultures and among girls of all economic backgrounds. The message is clear. Unlike little boys, who learn that they must move to the sideline so the game can continue, little girls demonstrate at an early age, that their emotions and their actions are woven into life's tapestry in ways that connect them with others. Females carry a sense of responsibility about other people's feelings that can easily become out-of-proportion and overshadow their accountability to their own wellbeing.

To make matters more complicated, neither genetic coding nor social mores have caught up with the way most women today live their lives. The roles of women have changed dramatically. Even though only one or two generations back, teen brides and teen mothers were common, women are now expected to accomplish a lot more before they settle into families of their own.

Men and women are living longer thanks to better health care and living conditions. Instead of fifty years to define a lifetime, women are living active, healthy lives into their seventies, eighties, even nineties. With nearly twice as much lifetime to fill with experiences, there also comes a greater timeframe for earning a living, accomplishing goals, and assuming responsibilities. Women work outside the home in record-high numbers, indirectly (and sometimes directly) challenging men to step up to the plate and assume more responsibility for child rearing and childcare.

As women's lives expand both in duration and in breadth of experiences, they now fulfill roles and expectations (their own and those of others) in ways no other generation has ever experienced. Demands come from every direction. Putting everyone else's needs first may have once ensured survival of the species, but these days, the scope of such demands may bury women before their time.

Putting yourself second to your mate and other individuals in your life may have worked in the past, but it does not work today. Just how unworkable it is, becomes dramatically apparent in the face of a life crisis such as infertility. In order to survive and thrive despite your infertility challenges, it is critical that you learn to say "yes," or to say "no," keeping in mind what is best for you. Making conscious choices that serve your own best interest does not mean you are selfish or self-centered. You can be a loving, generous woman, who also happens to make decisions based on whether they feel comfortable for you, rather than doing what you think others expect of you.

Sometimes the Right Thing Isn't What You Think It Is

Mary is one of Marina's clients. As with so many women, the idea of being *nice*, in Mary's mind, meant dismissing her own needs, and being accommodating to others. For three years, Mary and her husband, Kyle, tried to get pregnant, mostly on the high-tech track. Mary had unsuccessfully tried

IVF, both on her own and with an egg donor. As the ticking grew louder and louder on her biological clock, Mary found her coping skills taxed more and more, with her stress and frustration levels growing higher and higher.

Mary's emotions were already in overload when Kyle's lifelong best friend, Max, who lived several hundred miles away, called to ask if he, his wife Brenda, and their two-year-old daughter could come for a visit. Brenda and Max not only had one adorable little girl, but they could hardly contain their excitement over Brenda's pregnancy and the little boy due in only four months. Brenda was in exactly the place in her life that Mary wanted to be in hers. Even though Mary knew this, she wanted to be seen as a good sport, so she told Kyle (and herself) that the visit wouldn't really bother her. Mary overrode the doubts she felt and the clues her body was giving her, as she assured Kyle that she was fine with the upcoming visit.

Just after dinner on the first night of their stay, Mary ran to the store to pick up coffee creamer. When she returned to the house, the den and kitchen were empty. Climbing the stairs, Mary called everyone's name, wondering where the three friends had gone. Then she heard voices from the master bedroom.

Mary and Kyle's spacious master bedroom is really more of a suite, with two glass doors leading to an adjoining area—a room intended to be the nursery. The moment Mary stepped into her bedroom, she saw Kyle, Max, Brenda, and the two-year-old standing in what should have been her baby's nursery. Kyle and Max were assembling a crib in the room that had been empty, awaiting a baby to occupy it, for almost four years.

The scene Mary saw through the glass doors was her proverbial straw. Nice and accommodating fell by the wayside as Mary burst into tears and a stream of angry words she suddenly felt unable to stop. Brenda and Max, of course, felt terrible. Mary herself was both angry and embarrassed at the same time, and Kyle was uncomfortable for his friends, miserable to see his wife so distraught, and totally perplexed that Mary had told him she was

> ⊞ *nice and accommodating are not synonymous words*

okay with the visit when she so obviously was not okay at all.

"Nice" and "accommodating" are not synonyms. Mary was trying so hard to be nice in a way that was not required, that she never realized she had options. If Max and Brenda had stayed in a hotel, the two couples could have gotten together for dinner. Kyle and Mary could have even played tour guides to their city.

Mary did not need to see Max and Brenda—the happy fertile family—inside her own home. In fact, Mary's home could have and should have, remained her sanctuary, a place she could go to experience her emotions in private. If there were days during the visit that Mary did not feel up to socializing, she could have bypassed the outings with Max and Brenda entirely.

Instead, Mary invited Max and Brenda into her home and into her daily routine because she wanted to be seen as a good sport, likeable, amenable to the wants and requests of others. She ranked what Max and Brenda might think about her (and perhaps what she thought Kyle might think as well) ahead of what she thought about herself. She tried to control their response to her by giving them what she thought they wanted. But this type of giving is not clean. It doesn't come from a place where giving makes others happy *and* brings you joy. As a result, it backfired.

Do you see how differently the situation would have been for Mary if she had taken the time to think matters through, acknowledge her genuine emotions, and then do what was best for her? She could have avoided events that turned out to be painful for her and everyone involved. All four adults would have benefited from Mary's self-honesty.

Communication that Misses the Mark

There is a lot of wisdom in the adage, "We teach people how to treat us." You communicate with your world all the time and much of that communication has nothing to do with what you say. One well-known study conducted at UCLA determined that as much as ninety-three percent of communication is non-verbal. Some of the messages and signals you send to others are overt messages and some are subtle. In fact, in addition to the verbal communications you have and the boundaries you set with others, (which are discussed in Chapters 5 and 6) the most significant way you let other people know how you want to be treated is by *the way you treat yourself.*

Imagine that your relationship with yourself provides the template the rest of the world follows in determining how to behave toward you. If you treat yourself with honor and respect, (emotionally, spiritually, physically) you are letting everyone know that this is what you expect. In essence, you are setting the standard.

As the previous chapter explained, the simplest, most obvious place to begin the process of self-care is by taking care of your body. Making the choice to treat your body well, despite the fertility challenges you may be facing, is a meaningful, proactive decision. Caring for your physical self changes the way you see yourself, and provides a powerful communication to you and to others that you are a person of value. From there, it is a short step to making the emotional choices that best serve your life.

> ...the most significant way you let others know how you want to be treated is by the way you treat yourself

When you are demonstrably able to treat yourself well, you will start to live your life in a way that reinforces the process of making choices that are the best for you, instead of the choices you think are best for others. Your body and your mind will begin to work together to facilitate decisions that serve your total wellbeing.

Bear in mind, *you teach people how to treat you.* By not checking in with her own emotions and not acting on her authentic feelings in a forthright way, Mary was teaching her husband that it was okay to expect her to go along with things, even though this made her uncomfortable. To add to the confusion of her message, her choices and actions also taught him that despite the fact she said she was okay, he couldn't count on her words. She was teaching her husband to be apprehensive of the possibility that she might surprise him by reacting in ways that were incongruent with what she told him. Just as importantly, Mary was reinforcing to herself that her own feelings should take second place to what she perceived were the feelings of others.

There is no doubt that empathy is a positive quality. But as a woman, you need to be aware that empathy also carries the risk of losing yourself in the collectiveness of your relationships with others. For example, when Mary finally took the time to reflect on her situation in therapy, she realized her fatal flaw was that she had not checked in with herself and listened to her authentic feelings. If she had, she would have recognized that maybe just having dinner with her husband's friends would have been enough. Mary's feelings may have been difficult for her to read, yet her body, no doubt, was giving her indicators that would have made her feelings crystal clear. But first, Mary had to tune in to her internal communication and learn to read her own body's signals.

The "V" Word

The "V" word—vulnerability—has gotten a bad rap in recent years. People perceive vulnerability as a weakness; as leaving yourself unprotected and open to attack, *and heaven help you if you do that!*

Marina tells clients that vulnerability is strength—at which point, they often look at her as if she has grown another head! But think about this: when you are vulnerable, you are allowing yourself to really get in touch with your emotions. In allowing yourself to experience how you genuinely feel, (your authentic feelings of joy, sadness, and fear, for example) you place yourself in a position to make choices that serve *you,* and that are consistent with your needs and desires.

Look at Heidi, for example. Struggling to get pregnant, Heidi came into Marina's office complaining that it was increasingly difficult for her to socialize with her best friend, now that her friend was pregnant. Heidi rationalized that she had no right to feel the way she did, and tried to talk herself out of her feelings. To her, it felt weak to be so upset, because she reasoned, her friend had done nothing deliberately to hurt her.

Despite the fact that Heidi kept trying to talk herself out of her feelings, the knot in her stomach told her that these emotions just weren't going away. To make matters more complicated, rather than talking about her feelings directly, Heidi found herself acting them out, dodging phone calls from her friend, or making excuses to avoid getting together.

One day, Heidi realized she could no longer continue the charade. "It just became too much work to keep pretending," Heidi related. "So I took a deep breath, invited her to lunch, and just shared—from my heart—everything I was feeling. I told her how much I cared about her, how happy I was for her, but how hard it was for me to be around her right now. I let her know how scary it was to even be bringing this up, and my deep fear that we'd drift apart now that this separated us."

Heidi's candor may have surprised her friend, but in fact, it served as a testimony to their friendship. Heidi actually showed more respect for her friend, their relationship, and most importantly, herself, by being honest. Just avoiding her friend and not explaining the true reason why was actually a *disrespectful* way to handle the situation.

For Heidi, being vulnerable and admitting how she really felt, and then accepting the outcome her honesty would create, took a lot of strength. Nevertheless, doing so allowed her to make conscious choices about how she could move forward with the relationship, while still honoring her own emotions.

Letting Emotions Serve You, Not Enslave You

You knew that popular girl in high school. She rode the waves of her emotions in a very public way and she took as many others along with her as she could pull into the undertow. If she had a new crush, a fight with another girl, trouble with a teacher, or her parents lowered the boom on her, everyone in school knew about it. She was exuberant; she was heartbroken; she was humiliated, but she was never passive or private. When drama wasn't happening, she instigated it. She was a victim of her emotions, except because she was fifteen or maybe sixteen years young, she exploited her emotions as a way to draw attention to herself.

You are not sixteen and you hopefully have outgrown any need to be that high school drama queen. You no longer have to fear your emotions or to serve them. In fact, the reverse is true. Your emotions exist to serve you—they allow you to discover what is right for you. When you remember that you are experiencing certain feelings, but that *your feelings do not define you,* it becomes possible for you to stand apart from your emotions and in a sense, to watch them with curiosity, and use them to guide you in a positive way.

Start with the strong, nurtured, physical being you are creating by loving and caring for your body. As you become better at breathing right side up, instead of upside down, your emotional self will become a natural part of you, and a valuable and accessible part of your whole being. Your first thought may be, "Wait, I am already emotional enough right now. I can't deal with more emotions!" But breathing into your emotions will not cause you to experience *more* emotions. Breathing into yourself will allow you to process and move through what you are already feeling, so that you can make appropriate, mature decisions that work for you.

As you come to understand how your body responds to your emotions, you will begin to use these responses as your guide. In as much as your relationship with yourself is a template to the rest of the world for how to treat you, your body's responses to different types of situations and experiences become a template for you to use in decision-making.

It seems almost instinctive for many women that, as soon as a big feeling comes along, you immediately begin to hold your breath, literally choking back the feeling. When you do this, the very emotions meant to inform you and to support you, create a logjam of angst that blocks all positive movement in life. You literally lose access to a critical part of you, the part that provides direction and guidance.

When you breathe into your emotions, you acknowledge them and are able to notice how your body is responding. From there, it is a short step to realizing that choices need to be made, conscious choices, which honor and respect what you now know to be true for you.

Chapter 3 described effective breathing techniques that allow you to become aware of how you feel and how your body experiences your emotions. By breathing into your emotional sensations, you learn to move toward a greater conscious awareness of your

your emotions exist to serve you — they allow you to discover what is right for you

feelings. The body becomes a mechanism that allows you to tune in to your feelings. Becoming aware of your true emotions about making certain decisions is critical—it is the portal through which you must pass in order to determine whether something is right or wrong for you. Becoming more aware of your feelings is the *most direct route* to the skill of making conscious choices—those decisions that are genuinely right for you.

Partners in Conscious Choices

The body and the mind work as partners in allowing you to make the choices that serve you best. When you have a feeling, whether it is because you are experiencing something in the moment, or you are remembering something from the past, you experience that emotion with both your body and your mind. To see how this works, try the following simple exercise.

Close your eyes and imagine a time in your past when you faced a fork in the road and you had to make a decision about which way to go. Recall a choice that turned out well. Let yourself sit with this memory for a moment. Experience the jubilation of having made the right decision and the relief you felt when you realized things had turned out well. Breathe into this memory and notice: what is happening in your body? Do you see any changes, subtle or significant? Is there a warm feeling in the center of your body? A feeling of relaxation? Lightness in your head and shoulders? Does it have a certain quality—open and airy, sharp or dull? Does it stay in just one position, or does it move around? As you do this, don't attempt to change your experience in any way. Just watch it with a sense of wonder—watch and feel what is happening.

What you are experiencing in your body is a *felt sense* of your memory, of your emotional experience. Eugene Gendlin originally coined this term in his book, *Focusing*. He explained that a felt sense is not a mental experience—you are not analyzing or explaining what's happening. Instead, you are just getting quiet and being with a felt sense of your body's experience, or in Gendlin's words, "a bodily awareness of a situation, a person, or an event," either now, in the past, or in anticipation of some upcoming event.

Now try the process again. This time, imagine a choice you made in which the outcome was not what you had hoped it would be. Perhaps you chose a certain fertility treatment that met with a negative pregnancy result, or you decided to attend a baby shower and found your time there was difficult and upsetting. Notice now what your body is feeling: is there tightness in your chest? Heaviness in your heart? Butterflies in your stomach? Is there a specific quality to the feeling, like sticky, scary, or sad? Does it stay in one spot or does it move around? Again, be curious and just notice.

Even though these situations happened in the past, you can see how your body still has a memory of these experiences and the bodily feelings tied to them. Your mind can play tricks on you—it can rationalize, deny, or minimize certain feelings. But your body? It remembers, and it does not lie.

Your body can provide you with information, not only about previous experiences, but about where you are in the moment, as well. Say for example, like Heidi, you have been forcing yourself to go along with a situation that no longer serves you. Checking in with your body allows you to notice the knot in your stomach or the tension in your chest. Your body will alert you when you neglect your own emotional wellbeing in the choices you make, and when there is something you need to say or do for yourself. "Checking in" and becoming familiar with this felt sense of your body will tell you volumes about how you really feel, and what conscious choices would serve you best.

The Body Speaks

Even though each person's body is unique and has a language of its own, there are some general rules that apply and can be immensely helpful in understanding what your body is communicating. Research conducted at the Hendricks Institute and documented in *The Ten Second Miracle: Creating Relationship Breakthroughs* by Dr. Gay Hendricks, found that there are primarily three body zones, each with a specific "feeling" language all its own.

Zone 1 is your upper back, shoulders, neck, up into the jaw, and head. Tension and constriction here often communicates or represents anger, frustration, or aggravation.

Zone 2 is in the throat and chest. You may experience this tension as a lump in your throat, or tightness, constriction, or heaviness in the chest. This part of the body communicates sadness, hurt, and longing.

Zone 3 is the stomach and may present itself in the form of butterflies, or a racy, queasy feeling. This represents fear, anxiety, and nervousness.

Emotions help prepare your body for different types of physical responses. For example, there is a purposeful reason you lift your eyebrows when you are surprised. Lifting your brows physically lifts the eyelid thereby increasing your field of vision and giving you more information about the moment. When you grow pale with fear, it is physiologically because the emotion of fear reroutes blood flow from your face and head and directs it toward the large muscles in the legs and arms. Keep in mind, fear in your primitive brain means that you may need to fight or take flight.

Bodily reactions to your emotional state happen naturally and involuntarily. If you know how to read your body and to recognize *how* and *where* your body responds to emotions, you have access to a powerful piece of information to help you get in touch more accurately with your authentic emotions. Even during times you are not thinking clearly enough to discern your true feelings about something, you can still learn to identify the feeling by reading your own physical clues. Reread this section if you are not clear about this message; this is very important information. You never again have to say, "I don't *your body remembers and it does not lie* know how I feel" about something, if you learn how to read the messages your body so clearly communicates to you. Knowing how you feel about something is powerful information that opens the door to making conscious choices.

Start With Your ABC's

Here is a simple way to remember the three steps that can lead you from acknowledgement to conscious choice:

A.   Acknowledge

As soon as you notice you are experiencing an emotion, stop for a moment and acknowledge it. Acknowledge what is happening in both your body and your mind. What thoughts are you thinking? How is your body experiencing these emotions?

B. Breathe

Pause and take a breath into your emotional experience. Using the breathing process to filter your emotions allows you a little space for both your body and your mind to register what is happening.

C. Choose

Consider how you want to deal with what is happening. Is it enough just to be aware of what you are feeling, or is there something you need to do or say that will support you?

The second Power Tool, "Make Conscious Choices," serves as a bridge, connecting your awareness of your emotional self to the power you have to make choices. This bridge functions to acknowledge you, and allows you to make decisions that are right for you.

Try It On for Size

Correct breathing is a way to help you process your emotions. Breathe in, fully and deeply, the way a baby breathes. As you do, you will be unable to stop the emotion that washes over you like a wave.

The visual of a wave is a very good analogy for the way emotions are processed. When you experience a feeling and you breathe into it, your perception of it may get bigger as the emotion comes into your conscious awareness. Like a wave, the emotion then recedes once you've paid attention to it. Its work is done. Your emotion has informed you.

But once you've permitted the full scope of an emotion into your conscious self, *what do you do with that emotion?*

You try it on for size. The first and most essential step in making conscious choices is literally to "try it on." Instead of thinking of the emotion as something ethereal or intangible, give it a concrete form. You have your wool sweater, your tan SUV, your shelf of paperback books, and oh yes, you have that feeling that comes every time you think about your sister-in-law's upcoming baby shower.

Instead of just expecting to immediately know whether to attend the shower, (or any other choice or decision that needs to be made) give yourself the opportunity to sit with your feelings and to be open to the wisdom of your body. How do you really feel about moving forward in fertility treatment, continuing certain relationships, or attending an upcoming event? If you allow yourself to be vulnerable, to breathe and be open to the wisdom of your body, your emotions will guide you in making your choices.

As you first read this, you may think that you know the difference in the feeling of a good choice and the negative reaction that accompanies a bad choice. When it comes to all those events in life that are clearly black and white, those that are obviously a good choice or obviously a poor choice, then yes, you do recognize easily how to qualify such decisions as either right for you or wrong for you. However, very few aspects of infertility are easily categorized as black or white.

Many of the choices you must make during this time are not either obviously a good choice for you or a poor one. *Do I try IVF? Do I stop treatments now? Do I consider adoption?* These are tough questions and there is rarely a single correct answer to any of them. Remembering this is critical because sometimes you deceive yourself into thinking that there is a "right" choice out there. You wind up exhausting yourself trying to find out what that is. The truth is, there is no absolute right choice, only one that is best for you. In order to make the choices that are best for you, you need all the help you can get to understand what "best" really is.

we love to divide feelings, into categories but the truth of the matter is that feelings are not good or bad... they just are

The more conscious you are of the physical changes manifested because of your choices, the more easily you will recognize the feel of options that are a good fit for you and those that are not. This is particularly true in matters of infertility. As Jean and Michael Carter point out in their book, *Sweet Grapes, How to Stop Being Infertile and Start Living Again,* "...infertility can convince you into thinking that you have lost control of your body, and even your life. All you have to do is participate in fertility treatment to be reminded that you lack control." Being fully aware of your feelings and making conscious choices is a way for you to take back your power—to remember that you are in charge, and that ultimately, you and only you have the power to decide how you want to move forward.

Get Real

As you start to make conscious choices, be realistic about what you can handle. Respect yourself enough to do what works for you. For some of you, this may represent quite a turnaround in the way you've operated in the world so far. You may have to stop putting your time into commitments that no longer bring you joy, or for which you have no energy right now. You may choose to turn down invitations to events such as baby showers, or to curtail socializing with pregnant friends. Practice turning down invitations to things that you just don't feel like you can emotionally handle right now, or if you must attend, arrive late and leave early.

There is no right or wrong here; there is only what is best for you at this time. Developing the ability to acknowledge and respect your feelings, and acting accordingly, is a skill that will benefit you for the rest of your life. Likewise, it will benefit your spouse, your marriage, your friends, family, and everyone who cares about how you feel. The people you may be so concerned about protecting are also concerned about you. They would not want you to do things that make you uncomfortable or more stressed than you already are—if only you will communicate to them what those stress-makers are. Of course, you can only communicate what you genuinely want and need if you are able to recognize and take honest ownership of it yourself.

The challenge in being honest with yourself comes when you resist what you are feeling or what you want, because it does not measure up to an idealized view of yourself. Know that the tyranny of this perfection exists only in your mind, and you *can* choose to let it go. You are human! Accept that you have some feelings, and that some of these are not going to be consistent with your previous view of yourself. For example, you might find yourself jealous of a pregnant friend or a new mother. You also might find yourself feeling impatient with people who don't seem to understand what you're going through. People love to divide feelings into categories rationalizing that happy is a good feeling and anger or fear are bad feelings. Keep reminding yourself, feelings are not good or bad—they just are.

Good or bad comes in to play because of what you do with your feelings and how you act them out. It is okay and it is normal to feel jealousy or resentment. What is not okay is to act out your feelings in a hurtful way. This means that you don't want to treat someone unkindly because she is pregnant and you are not. You must acknowledge that "hurtful" applies to self-hurt in the same way it applies to hurting others. Do not put yourself in a position to feel more pain as part of a misdirected effort to do the right thing. Do what feels most comfortable for you, but be candid with the other people involved.

Even if you have always been the one who acquiesces to the needs or demands of others, don't lose sight of the fact that no personality trait or pattern has to be a permanent part of who you are. Change can be very difficult to make, but it is achievable. The very fact that you go through your life with the freedom to change, grow, and redefine yourself is one of the most exciting things about being human. Unlike other creatures on this planet, you have the opportunity consciously to choose and consciously to create a life that works for you.

Women may be cast into roles at an early age and then no matter how old they become, how much they achieve, or how far away they travel, they carry those personas, like characters in a play, along with them. But when you learn to send different messages to people, you will find that they are aware of you and respond to you in different ways. Despite the fact that you were labeled as the shy child, the talkative girl, or the aggressive businesswoman, if it is a title you don't feel comfortable wearing, you have the power to reprogram the message you send to the world. When you send a different message, the world will begin to treat you in a different way. As this starts to happen, you will also find that you begin to treat yourself differently. No matter where you are in life, you are never too young, too old, or too set in your ways to make positive life changes. Oftentimes, the trauma of a life crisis like infertility is exactly what you need to spur such a transformation.

Most people are aware that in the aftermath of a destructive forest fire, which may leave hundreds, perhaps thousands of acres blackened and seemingly devoid of all life, always—one hundred percent of the time—

there follows a period of abundant, flourishing growth. What grows on the charred forest floor is not the same as what grew there before the fire, yet the new growth is strong, verdant, and plentiful.

As burned-out as your infertility struggle may leave you, it does provide you that perfect opportunity for positive change. In this regard, your fertility challenges come with the "gift" of giving you the chance to learn how to be true to yourself.

Look back at how many times you have done what was right for someone else at the expense of what your heart (or your gut) told you to do. Wouldn't it be wonderful to break free of that type of decision-making? Wouldn't it be incredible to be able to be true to your authentic self, not just during this time, but for the rest of your life? Your experience with infertility can offer you this watershed opportunity. You can broaden your self-image by being willing to embrace yourself as a woman who is loving, generous, and willing to say "yes" or "no" with your own wellbeing as the priority. Chapter 6, "Telling the Truth," will help you polish your new skills in communicating with others more authentically, by giving you language that actually equips you to tell your own truth.

Over time, medical science may or may not change your fertility situation. Perhaps that door in your life has already closed. If you are currently involved in treatment, you know that beyond maintaining optimal physical and mental health and cooperating with the regimens of fertility treatments, you can do relatively little to change your fertility. You cannot change the outcome of procedures you may undergo, the costs of the treatments, or the options fertility research gives you.

But you can change how you choose to respond to each element of your situation. You can change the relationship you are creating with yourself along the way. When all is said and done, how you emerge from this, and who you become because of this experience, is something that will either enhance or diminish you for the rest of your life. You get to decide who you will be. Don't miss this opportunity to learn to check in with your body and your mind, with the emotions that are housed there, and then, from that place, to make conscious choices to support all of your decisions.

FROM MARINA'S CASE FILE ON

Lucinda R.

*L*ucinda represents the transition that can occur when a life crisis, like infertility, invites you to take off the mask of who you pretend to be, and expose the raw and powerful vulnerability underneath the pretense. As you'll see with Lucinda, one conscious choice can open the door to the next.

Lucinda is a thirty-two year old woman who has been in fertility treatment for the past two years, most recently having undergone her first IVF, which was unsuccessful. She states that her husband is loving and supportive and, other than her struggle with fertility issues, she sees herself as content with her life. Lucinda is bright and successful, and a few years ago broke off from her parent company to start her own advertising firm. The hours are long and work is hard, she tells me, but she enjoys what she does. But despite her career success, Lucinda revealed that "just being a mom" is what she's always really wanted to do. Lucinda's mother was a stay-at-home mom, and she has always envisioned herself creating the same great memories with her own children.

Ironically, Lucinda revealed that part of the reason for her career success is that she is at the age where all her friends are now settling down and having babies. This has been painful for her, but since she has never been one to appear vulnerable, she has ramped up the "corporate success" persona, pretending that her difficulty having children is really a choice to be childfree for now. Lucinda's M.O. has been to, "never let them see you sweat," and she acknowledges that she even emotionally withholds to her mother and her husband. Now, however, she is finding that the strain of pretending is becoming too emotionally difficult.

When Lucinda first enters treatment, she finds herself exploring her fears around being authentic, and how abandoning a personality that has been built on being an achiever and being in control, is terrifying to her. She is so closely identified with this way of being, that she finds it hard to imagine that there's anything of value underneath. Despite this, she can't help but acknowledge the physical tension and emotional toll these personas have caused, so, in a leap of faith, she takes her first step. She learns to breathe properly, and in so doing, opens the door to letting herself actually feel.

As she opens to her world of feelings, Lucinda yearns for additional tools to help her to "be with" the emotions of her emerging self. She begins to journal and to meditate. As she does, she realizes that it now becomes necessary to express to others the truth she is discovering about herself. She learns ways to educate her husband and mother about what she needs, rather than pretend everything is fine in order to protect them.

In the interim, Lucinda continues to undergo fertility treatment, vacillating from hope to disappointment, compounded by the side effects of the fertility medication. But despite all this, she starts to feel better, "more like herself." She learns to recognize core feelings, and begins to make choices that feel right for her, as opposed to the image she wants to project. Most importantly, she becomes involved in a local fertility support group, and there meets women who are "just like her," and who can provide her with the safety and understanding she needs. Her new experiences and new network of support allow her to become more truthful with old friends, and she begins to share the story of her struggle, and take space from social interactions, like child-centered events, that seem just too painful for her right now.

Over time, Lucinda begins to acknowledge that continuing in her high-powered executive position is causing too much stress in her life. In addition, she becomes concerned that this is working against her in her goal of becoming pregnant. So, after much discussion, she decides to hand over the reins of her company, and become a full-time homemaker. She begins her second cycle of IVF, while mourning her former life, and old ways of validating her self-worth. This is a tough transition, but, slowly, she explores new outlets for herself. She gets involved in her community, she starts a garden, she takes long walks…in short, she begins to build the life about which she has always dreamed.

Finally, on her third attempt at IVF, Lucinda becomes pregnant with her daughter. But, she acknowledges, this experience has been about a lot more than just being able to have a baby. On her last session she marvels that this journey has really taken her home to herself—and that the person she has discovered herself to be is so much more than who she thought she was.

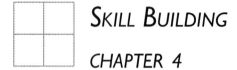

SKILL BUILDING

CHAPTER 4

In science, the litmus test is a simple examination that uses specially treated papers which, when exposed to a liquid, immediately tell the viewer if the liquid is acid or alkaline and to what degree. To ensure that you make your wellbeing a top priority in the choices you make, use the following questions as your litmus test through which you filter your experiences.

1. Before you say "yes" to something that may make you uncomfortable or simply not be right for you, ask yourself the following questions:

    Will this or does this bring me joy?

    Is this what I would like to do?

    How would I like this to be done?

    How would I like this situation to be?

2. Now look at what is already in place in your life. Ask yourself:

    Are my choices working for me?

    What can I say "no" to that I have already said "yes" to?

    Is there a way to honor my feelings, while still keeping a commitment?

    If I want to break this commitment, how can I do it responsibly?

    How can I get comfortable with just saying "no"?

3. If there are areas of your life that are particularly challenging in terms of
    determining what choice is right for you, look again at the case study of
    Lucinda R. Notice the choices she made in an effort to project a certain
    image, such as, "super achiever," or "in control," and then, look at the
    transition she made as her choices began to go beyond these personas,
    and reflect her authentic self. Now ask yourself if some of your struggle is
    due to your resistance to giving up a certain persona, and taking a risk to
    express who you really are.

Your Third Power Tool: Set Healthy Boundaries

When you pack your toolbox with new life skills, you empower yourself not to merely get through your fertility challenges, but to come out of the experience as a better, stronger woman. As part of this learning, you will quickly discover that developing the ability to set healthy boundaries will serve you as one of your most beneficial tools. Healthy boundaries do not stand alone. In fact, this skill builds on, and is an extension of, making conscious choices.

As you have already learned, making conscious choices occurs when you check in with yourself and you are honest about how you feel and what you need. The next tool, setting healthy boundaries, builds upon that process by helping you develop skills to take care of yourself while you are in relationships with others. Unless you can identify where to draw the lines of healthy boundaries, it can be very difficult to understand where you stop and others begin, or more specifically, to know how taking care of yourself fits into being there for other people. Learning to set healthy boundaries allows you to clarify this so you can still be in relationships

your third power tool is: set healthy boundaries

with others while taking care of your genuine needs. Healthy boundaries do not test or strain your connections with others; instead, they strengthen them.

The first challenge of setting healthy boundaries comes with the word, healthy. Most people find it amazingly easy to create less-than-healthy ways to interact with others. Because of this, it is important to understand up front what boundaries are, and the balance that is necessary to create them.

If physical walls surround a country, that country does not have a functional or healthy boundary. A country separated from its neighbors, and from the rest of the world, is a police state, a prison that locks the citizens inside and prevents healthy interaction with people on the other side. But as harmful as it is to build walls around a country, it is just as detrimental if a country has no boundaries at all. Absence of boundaries allows anyone or anything to enter the country, even elements that could be hazardous to the citizens inside. A country needs to have, and benefits from having, *clearly defined* boundaries. By delineating their boundaries and educating other people about the terms and guidelines for crossing the boundaries, both the people on the inside and the people on the outside of a country are protected. Both gain. There are no secrets or hidden agendas—just clarity about what it takes to leave or to gain access.

Like an isolated country, if you build walls in your relationships with others, the walls alienate you and prevent you from dealing with important issues. Walls trap you and distance you from other people and from your own goals. Walls stand between you and the benefits you could gain from the people who care about you and should be part of your support system.

When your personal boundaries are well-marked and functional fences, they protect you. A good boundary defines your edge, that limit that separates you from others. For example, your skin is a boundary, with everything inside the skin being the physical you, and everything on the outside being the rest of the world. If you have an injury to your skin, a cut or scratch, you become more vulnerable to infection. As Anne Katherine discusses in her book, *Boundaries: Where You Begin and I End,* in much the same way, if your emotional boundaries are trespassed upon by the insensitive or intrusive actions of others, you also become susceptible to harm. Healthy boundaries create safety and serve to enhance your wellbeing.

Robert Frost said, "Good fences make good neighbors." Good fences are an excellent way to think about boundaries because not only do fences include gates that can be opened and closed, but it is also possible to see over and through fences. This allows you to know what is coming and what is around you, so that you make choices that work for you. You can keep out the people, places, and circumstances that don't serve you, and you can let in those that do. You are the gatekeeper. Healthy boundaries allow you to care for yourself, while being in relationships with others. And like fences, good boundaries have to be maintained—you need to keep paying attention to what you're allowing in and out of your life, so that you can continue to take care of yourself.

> *healthy boundaries allow you to care for yourself while being in relationships with others*

Walls Keep the Bad Stuff In

Chapter 1 includes words that are very hard to hear: *the baby is not the prize.* The rationale for this statement is simple. If your struggle to conceive has caused underlying problems to come to the surface, having a baby will not automatically make these issues go away. Having a baby will cure the matter of childlessness. But as for giving you the perfect life, fixing the problems in your relationships, making your happy if you are not, and all those other issues—well, they have to be addressed on their own.

A popular talk show aired a segment on women who had gone to great extremes to lose massive amounts of weight. The women had resorted to more than diet and exercise in order to achieve their weight loss; they had undergone gastric bypass surgery to diminish surgically the size of their stomachs. Sadly, the women later discovered that shedding the pounds and being thin did not solve anything. Yes, it put an end to obesity and the weight loss itself improved their appearance and improved their health. But when interviewed, the women stated that the weight loss, in and of itself, *did not make them happier.* The demons that haunted them before the surgery, such as lack of self-confidence, anger about their childhood, or fear of rejection, were all still alive and well inside the walls that surrounded their lives.

Unlike Jan from Chapter 1, who saw her struggles with infertility as an opportunity to deal with deeper issues and create a personal breakthrough, these women did not see their obesity as representing the wall that was obstructing their overall progress in life. They ended up with a new dress size, but they missed the opportunity to use their challenge as a time for problem solving and growth.

In these cases of weight-loss-gone-wrong, the problem started with the fact that being overweight was not the problem. Being overweight was only a symptom of a deeper issue. Certainly sometimes, there is a metabolic reason for excessive weight gain, but in most cases of obesity, the weight is the result of overeating, binge eating, or an unhealthy lifestyle, which is indicative of a deeper issue. Obesity is only a symptom of a more profound crisis.

So what's the connection between overeating and a true medical condition like infertility? How can there possibly be a parallel between eating too much food and wanting to conceive a sweet baby? Unfortunately, there is.

Facing fertility challenges without experiencing sadness, disappointment, frustration, and a host of other emotions is impossible. But when these feelings take over your life—when you become defined in your own mind by your infertility in such a way that it deeply impacts your relationship with yourself and others—then the emotions you are dealing with are symptomatic of other problems as well. Infertility related issues are some of the hardest to work through because the desire to have a child has roots that go all the way down to the coding in your DNA that tells you to reproduce.

Fitting into a size 8 dress does not fix all the things in life that an overweight woman may expect it to fix. Buying a bigger, better home does not fix problems in a troubled marriage and having a baby will not put your life back into balance if the challenges of infertility have brought to light problems that already existed or issues that needed to be addressed.

As you build boundaries to help you deal with fertility challenges, you must be very careful that you are building fences to let in what works for you and keep out what doesn't, but that you are not building walls. Not having boundaries at all would leave you defenseless and unprotected, but building walls only serves to isolate you. For example, if you find that in your grief, you are emotionally "bleeding" all over others in a way that doesn't respect their limits, and doesn't acknowledge where you end and they begin, then that's a problem. On the other hand, if you find that you are handling your grief by disconnecting and cutting yourself off from

⊞ *good boundaries restore flexibility and wholeness*

the support of others, that too is a concern. Each polarity represents the possibility you are playing out old patterns in ways that do not serve you. Here is a valuable clue that you might be doing exactly that: beware any time you have emotional déjà vu!

When you were dating, you may have experienced the feeling of becoming involved with the same man over and over again, even though it was really a series of men. Or, maybe you were attracted to someone who on the surface seemed different from the others, but within a surprisingly short period of time, you ended up feeling in your new relationship much like you had in the other relationships. Like magnets, women often are attracted to the same type of man, repeatedly. One theory is that people are attracted to a potential partner who represents the opportunity to successfully complete unfinished business from their childhood, usually business dealing with one parent or the other. In other words, the person who catches your eye may ignite in you a familiar sense of longing to do, or have, or feel in ways that escaped you as a child. It's like some unconscious part of you is saying, "Well, I couldn't get my father's attention or my mother's approval when I was a kid…and there's something about this person that triggers that same yearning, that same feeling, so I'm going to try again. Who knows—this time, I might get it right!"

The expression, "you complete me" may sound terribly romantic, but, as anyone on the other side of a broken love affair can tell you, two incomplete people really do not make a healthy whole. After all, how much difference is there between "he needs me" and "he's needy"? Any time you have challenging people in your life, whether they are your mate, your friend, or your boss, and who are so much like your last challenging mate, friend, or boss; you should read this as a big clue that you might be repeating old patterns because of unsolved issues in your own existence.

Wherever You Go, There You Are

Relationships that did not work out before are not going to work out this time just because the names and faces change. It may be tempting to think that the problem is your partner or your friend, and that all you have to do is dump him or her to be free of the problem. The truth is however, that unless you examine what it is about you that keeps recreating this, you'll continue to meet yourself and your familiar patterns in every new relationship. In the wise words of poet Edna St. Vincent Millet, "It's not true that life is one damn thing after another; it's one damn thing over and over again."

These types of relationships are interesting because they not only draw you to what is familiar; they also provide the opportunity for you to play a role or persona you know so well. For example, Alicia was a caregiving daughter to an unstable mother, and as an adult, found herself drawn to relationships that allowed her again to play the role of caregiver. Without consciously realizing it, she was attracted to needy people, and was always the first to lend a hand in any situation. When she first met Eddie, Alicia admired his independence and self-reliance. Unlike other relationships she had, Eddie proved he was capable of taking care of himself—a real bonus in her eyes, especially since she was still caring for her elderly mother.

Still, Alicia was intimately familiar with the role of caregiver and it formed the basis for how she "did" all relationships. As a result, she found herself catering to Eddie's every need, every request—real or imagined. Conditioned from childhood to be a caregiver, Alicia would just jump right in, anticipating, doing, taking care of, until finally, Eddie became dependent upon her always being there. At first this seemed like a marriage made in heaven, and with primarily Eddie and her mother in her life to tend to, Alicia managed quite well. The fact that she never reached out or acknowledged what she needed, was not *yet* a problem.

Then came the slam of infertility, with its seemingly incessant stream of doctor's appointments, testing, and emotional strain. In typical style, at first Alicia juggled it all, making all the arrangements and keeping her emotional struggle to herself. Soon Alicia grew exhausted with putting herself last and just doing, doing, doing for Eddie, her mother, and everyone else. The persona of caregiver that had carried her through life this far, that gave her meaning and purpose, was now turning against her. She needed to learn new skills that allowed her to discover ways to take care of herself *while* she was in relationships with other people. Essentially, she needed to learn to set healthy boundaries.

Even though there is nothing wrong with being a caregiver *when it's appropriate,* personas like the caregiver become problematic when they turn into masks behind which you hide your true feelings from others and from yourself. For example, if you find yourself thinking, "Well, if I'm not taking care of people, I'm not sure who I am or what value I'd have," you must stop and reassess the roles you have been playing. Despite the fact that there is a great deal of socialization and even a measure of inherent biology in the tendency of women to act as caregivers, a healthy life is about balance, about knowing when to give, as well as when to ask for and receive what you need. When you act simply from the role of your assumed persona, there's rigidity, a sense of being compelled to play the role even though it is not working for you. When this happens, you have lost touch with the other options you have—you have lost touch with the *whole of you.*

Good boundaries restore flexibility and wholeness. Rather than reacting based on behaviors that you have used or defaulted to in the past, you are

free to do what's right in the moment. Good boundaries allow
you to reconnect with your sense
of wholeness by allowing you to
consciously step into whatever
role serves you and others best.

> *we have too little time to waste it in relationships that are not equal and mutually rewarding. exchanging energy nourishes our souls* — SUE PATTON THEOLE

Building walls instead of setting boundaries allows your old problems and negative patterns to thrive unchallenged. Even if your circumstances change, not addressing your underlying issues means that the patterns are likely to reappear in a new form. Like insidious, stubborn weeds among your flowers or that unhealthy black mold that grows in your shower, some things are ongoing battles in life. The problems you had before you faced infertility may have reemerged under your current stress, but they are not problems caused by this experience. Sadly, even giving birth to a biological child is not going to make such problems go away.

Infertility is a true life crisis. Like the death of a spouse or a diagnosis of illness, infertility brings into your life a type of pain that never totally ends. But infertility doesn't have to destroy or even define the rest of your existence, even though it *will* change it. One of your challenges in dealing with infertility is being able to separate the stress that is logically part of dealing with this crisis from those stresses that have grown out of other experiences and other issues in your life. Learning to build healthy boundaries makes it easier for you to do this, because the fences you are putting in place become an infrastructure for your overall psychological health and wellbeing. Like any other structure you might build, when you create a solid foundation, everything you build upon it is stronger.

When you were fourteen or maybe seventeen, there was a cute boy with incredible eyes, who no doubt, broke your heart. Few people reach adulthood without experiencing this type of pain. At the time, it seemed as though your world had ended and you would never get over your anguish, but as the weeks went by, you found that your heartbreak began to hurt in a different and less-painful way. The part of your life once filled by Jeff or Marty, after a while, began to be filled with other things. Sometimes it was a new boyfriend, but more often, it was a collective of new interests that filled the spaces that had previously housed your young romance. As hurtful as your heartbreak felt at the time, it probably served as a type of dress rehearsal for experiences that came later in life. You learned you could recover from painful events, loss, and circumstances that seemed overwhelming. You learned there was life after Jeff or Marty and you gained a point of reference for facing the next painful experience in your world.

Infertility hurts, and as you have already learned, it is often the first life crisis many women experience or that most married couples go through together. There is absolutely no way it is painless. Yet, as you move day to day through your fertility challenges, you can make your pain more manageable. You must differentiate the stress that is a realistic part of this experience from the stresses of old hurts and wounds that are rooted in something entirely different. In Chapter 8, you will learn how the power tool, "Give Yourself Permission to Grieve," can help you process your sorrow in ways that lead to healing and growth.

Walls Also Keep the Good Stuff Out

You may think walls can protect you, but in truth, walls confine you. Walls separate you from others, restrict your freedom, and limit your perspective about life and events. A client once explained how she set her version of boundaries in her life, "When I've had enough, I put up a wall to keep other people out."

Surprisingly, this is the way many women approach the matter of boundaries. They give and give, tolerate and tolerate, and then—frequently in an emotion-laden outburst—they break down. Remember Mary's temperamental eruption because she couldn't deal with her husband and his friends in the nursery she thought would already be home to her own child? You can fake it for only so long before you hit your breaking point. An explosion or an equally destructive implosion will always occur. A powerful question to ask yourself is, "What are you pretending not to know?"

Walls you put up because you "have had enough" are not healthy boundaries—they are futile attempts to cap off emotional overload. Whatever the issue is, it will always surface when you have faked it as long as you can and then reach the point of exhaustion.

You need to let certain people and certain experiences come through your gate. People who love and support you are on the top of the list. But people cannot get inside unless you share with them your truths. When you tell your friend you are having a rough time, and that you don't feel comfortable going to her baby shower, you are giving her the truth—like a ticket to pass through the gate you use to mark your boundary. Rather than pretending to be something you're not—faking it to play your persona of the "unselfish friend," for example, you are telling her the truth, and in the process, revealing the whole of yourself. Armed with information she can count on to be valid, your friend can now respond to you in ways that will support your needs and help you take better care of yourself.

A good way to think about setting healthy boundaries is in the context of taking responsibility for yourself. When you think of taking responsibility, you may think of obligations or even burdens—things you *have* to do. For example, "I have to clean the kitchen," or "I have to pick up the dry cleaning." But these are not examples of taking responsibility to set healthy boundaries; they are just "stuff" that makes up life.

Taking healthy responsibility means that you become *wholly responsible for yourself*. You make choices that foster your wellbeing, and you communicate clearly to those around you how you feel, what you need, and what you would like to see happen. You choose to express yourself as a whole person.

When you step into this type of responsibility, you relieve others in your life from any need to "carry" you emotionally. They can stop trying to guess what you want or need. Taking healthy responsibility also means that you see other people in your world as capable of making responsible choices about their own lives as well. They too, can choose to be whole—to take responsibility for themselves, and tell you what they need and how they feel.

Alicia, the classic caregiver, struggled with this concept of responsibility on both counts. In the first place, she dropped the ball in terms of being accountable for her own wellbeing. Since she was trapped in the role of a caregiver, Alicia stuffed her awareness of how she felt and what she needed. In fact, without consciously realizing it, Alicia had struck an unhealthy bargain with her world. The bargain worked something like this: "I'll take care of other people, and in return other people will appreciate me and need me, and make me feel good about myself. In this way, other people are responsible for taking care of my needs." Alicia's deal with life is representative of poor boundaries.

People, even those closest to you, cannot know what you need or how you feel. Remember how Chapter 1 pointed out that you can't expect your husband or partner to be a psychic intuitive? Your responsibility is to become aware of your own needs and then communicate them so that others know what you would like them to do and how you really need them to respond. In this way, you are taking care of yourself.

The second way Alicia was failing to set healthy boundaries was that she not only took care of her mother, who really did need her help; Alicia took care of *everybody*, including her husband who was perfectly capable of doing much more for himself. Rather than remembering what drew her to him to begin with, namely his self-reliance and independence, Alicia overstepped her role with Eddie, doing so many things for him that he began to lose sight of his own skills to take care of himself. Eddie became dependent and added unnecessarily to Alicia's already full plate.

Look at your own life. Are there places where you are taking on projects or obligations that do not belong to you, or could easily be done by someone else? Are you stuffing your own needs and feelings because you do not want to hurt someone else's feelings? Are you afraid to say no, believing your value lies only in you being there for others? Are you there for others in ways that are causing you to neglect yourself?

If overdoing for other people is going on in your life, you are out of balance in the responsibility arena, and you need to make some changes. You need to make changes, *not* because you are dealing with the stresses of infertility, but because changes are genuinely necessary in order to have a balanced, mentally healthy adult life. Infertility is providing the invitation to take these steps.

Who Stays and Who Goes

When you begin to take healthy responsibility for yourself and you start, for perhaps the first time in twenty, thirty, or even forty years, communicating honestly with other people, you are going to alter some of your relationships. You are going to shake up some of the people in your life.

When you begin to take responsibility for yourself, there will be some awkward moments and a few missed cues because you are interacting with

now is the perfect time in your life for you to begin to move away from draining or negative relationships

others in a way that will be different from how you have acted in the past. Friends with whom you share healthy relationships naturally will be surprised when you start communicating with them more honestly, but they will also appreciate it. The people you really want in your life will be glad to deal with you in a more straightforward way. Your healthy relationships will flourish because of your changes. There will also be those relationships that do not flourish; the positive changes you are making will threaten them. You will find some of your current relationships exist because you have been drawn to or have attracted certain types of people—people who are attached to the persona you are playing, but not the whole of who you are. This is the relationship déjà vu described earlier.

There will always be problems with relationships if you take too little responsibility for yourself *or too much responsibility for others.* As Gay and Kathlyn Hendricks discuss in their book, *Conscious Loving: The Journey to Co-Commitment,* relationship conflicts stem from an imbalance in responsibility. Now is the perfect time in your life for you to begin to move away from any draining or negative relationships.

Look candidly at the people in your circle of friends. Which friendships require inordinate nurturing and attention in order to survive? Which relationships make you feel tired or as if you can never do enough for that person, no matter how much you try? And which associations immediately begin to plummet as soon as you stop taking responsibility for the other person, and start thinking instead about what's right for you?

You have one life; one amazingly short life, probably made up of about 28,000 days. If you are thirty years old, nearly 11,000 of those days are already behind you. How many of the rest of your days are you willing to spend in relationships that drain your energy? For that matter, how many of the rest of your days are you going to abandon the whole of you, and deprive yourself of the support you need to get through the tough times, whether it is infertility or any other circumstance life hands you?

Your life crisis places you at a pivotal point in your existence. You cannot change the fact that infertility has become part of your world. You can only change how you experience this challenge. If you believe this is a horrible, unfair event in your life, from which you can never recover, then that is exactly what it will prove to be. On the other hand, if you believe your experience with infertility is both a huge, life-changing disappointment *and* an opportunity for personal breakthrough, then it will become the growth impetus you believe it to be.

Ask yourself why you may be hanging on to any friendship, any relationship, that is handing you more stress than happiness. Once you identify these unbalanced relationships, begin to move away from them. In many cases, as you redefine yourself as a person who takes responsibility for herself, some of your less healthy relationships will begin to fade on their own. Let them go. It really is okay to back away from and put less of your energy into these imbalanced associations. As you do this, you will create space, and open up your life to new, healthier, and more enriching friendships and acquaintances.

Have the courage to expand your circle. You may want to consider deliberately building new bonds with women who are happily childfree, whose children are already grown, or whose lives and whose conversations do not revolve entirely around their offspring. Why not choose to give yourself a break? Move away from the types of issues that are creating pressure or stress for you right now. Allow yourself to become more receptive to new friendships with women who have created families in ways other than giving birth to a biological child, or women who have fulfilled their lives by giving birth to a business, a career, or a rewarding hobby.

Raising flowers is never the same as raising children and climbing mountaintops is not like watching your child grow to adulthood, but women who cultivate exotic flowers or scale a challenging rock wall will tell you that they gain a different but valued form of satisfaction from their accomplishments. Your goal is not to alienate yourself from your friends with children, or even from other friends who similarly may be struggling to conceive. Rather, your goal is to open yourself up to also enjoying relationships with women who experience their lives in ways not defined by motherhood in the traditional sense.

As you create new friendships, use your new skills to take responsibility for yourself from the very beginning of the relationship. If the relationship grows, you can feel confident you are building a friendship that will prove to be both healthy and meaningful.

Healthy responsibility yields healthy boundaries. Likewise, healthy boundaries foster healthy relationships. Good boundaries always create safety and integrity. They allow you to come to terms with where you stand and what you need, and to make plans and take actions in your life that are consistent with those needs. Good boundaries create the strongest platform from which to build a good marriage, a meaningful career, mutually supportive friendships, and a life worth living every single day.

FROM MARINA'S CASE FILES ON
Sophia and Carlos W.

this case history demonstrates how much can be hidden under the diagnosis of infertility. In this situation, fertility treatment seemed just a cover for an absence of intimacy in the marriage, as well as a history of sexual abuse.

Sophia came to see me with a diagnosis of unexplained infertility. For the past year, the couple has been under the treatment of an infertility specialist and contemplating IVF. When Sophia shared her history initially in counseling, she appeared to be primarily dealing with issues of low self-esteem and feelings of unworthiness. Sophia shared that while she was in college, she had an abortion, and she believes she is being "punished by God," through her infertility. Although Sophia is of average height and weight, she sees herself as extremely unattractive. The roots of this, she says, are in her moralistic upbringing, as well as the hypercritical feedback she has always received from her father. Sophia also complains of lack of support from her husband, as well as his peripheral involvement in fertility treatment.

When Carlos tells his side of the story, he acknowledges that although his priorities in life are God, family, and work, the truth of his life evidences priorities of work, work, and work. He too, complains of a father-in-law who is too involved and too critical, and states that Sophia's vulnerability to this stresses her and their relationship. In particular, he complains of their lack of intimacy, in essence, a virtual absence of a sex life. He believes that Sophia is moving "too fast" to become involved in fertility treatment, and not giving "nature" a chance. He stated that although neither were virgins when they met one another, they decided to wait until they got married to have sexual relations. This part of their relationship has always been infrequent and unsatisfying, and he attributes this to Sophia's poor body image. Sophia concurs with this.

Treatment begins by working with Sophia to address these internalized, critical messages, as well as educating her in ways to set healthy boundaries with her father. In addition, Sophia also learns ways to ask specifically for what she wants and needs from Carlos. With clarity about how to be a supportive husband, Carlos becomes more willing to make efforts to balance work and home.

Despite these positive changes, and a more compatible marriage overall, their sexual relationship remains unchanged. This is confusing to Sophia who, as her self-esteem grows, makes an effort to be more responsive and available. Couples counseling is initiated, and Carlos becomes aware that even though he complains of a lack of intimacy in the marriage, he will often engage in the very behaviors that sabotage closeness. Despite this acknowledgement, however, Carlos was unwilling to make any changes in this pattern, and shortly thereafter, the couple decides to take a break from treatment.

They return to counseling about two years later. Since then, Sophia has undergone IVF, and given birth to a son. Again, the couple's presenting problem is Carlos's complaint of lack of intimacy. I follow a protocol that explores ways to be intimate, and begin assigning homework for the couple. Again, I notice that despite the fact that this issue has been historically regarded in the relationship as "Sophia's problem," Carlos subtly continues to sabotage closeness. During a couple's session, not only do I address this directly, but also I question Carlos's willingness to tolerate an absence of intimacy for months at a time. Carlos agrees to be seen individually and to explore the issue further. Over time, Carlos uncovers his own history of childhood sexual abuse by a close family friend, a prominent leader of the community's youth organization. Work begins in processing the shame and rage he has carried from this. As he heals, he is able to see how these incidents impacted his feelings about his own sexuality, and, of course, his unwillingness to be intimate with his wife.

When Carlos felt ready, their therapy as a couple was able to resume once again, and built on the foundation of their loving relationship, they were able to make great strides. At last report, Carlos and Sophia were enjoying all aspects of a loving and intimate relationship.

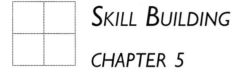

SKILL BUILDING

CHAPTER 5

The marriage of the couple in the case study used in Chapter 5, Sophia and Carlos W, is impacted by several instances of poor or crossed boundaries such as a lack of work-life balance, the over-involvement of a hypercritical mother, even a case of childhood sexual abuse. Although aspects of their situation may appear extreme to you, their situation can help you to understand the snowball effect of poor boundaries.

Now look at the boundaries in your life, and ask yourself: Where am I in relationship to everything else? Are there people or circumstances that are crowding me with demands? Am I isolating myself, or shutting down to my own needs? What choices can I make to start developing healthier boundaries that allow me to care for myself first?

Setting boundaries with people...

1. Sometimes you can see in others what you cannot see in yourself. List friends, coworkers, and family members you know that seem to say "yes" to everything; people who do not set healthy boundaries.

2. List the positive outcomes you see from their behavior. List the negative.

3. List friends, coworkers, and family members you know who seem to be comfortable with saying "no" to things that are not right for them; people who seem to be able to set healthy boundaries.

4. List the positive and negative outcomes you see from their behavior.

5. Now list specific things you can do to create healthier boundaries for yourself.

Setting boundaries with places and things...

6. Radio, TV, the news, traffic, just plain noise! Sometimes it's easy to feel bombarded from so much extraneous stimulation, especially when you're already dealing with a full plate. Take heart; even small decisions like not watching the news before bed, having a TV-free evening once a week, or leaving for work a little later or a little earlier in the morning in order to miss the traffic, can make a big difference. List four boundaries you can set with the "places and things" in your life, in order to create a calmer, less stressful lifestyle.

CHAPTER 6

Your Fourth Power Tool: Tell the Truth

Healthy boundaries happen when you tell the truth.
At first glance, you may find yourself a bit put off at this statement. "I don't lie," you may be thinking, "so I'm already practicing this tool." But the fourth power tool is about a different kind of
truthfulness than the way most people think of truth and lies. The truth
tool doesn't deal with concepts or opinions. Telling your best friend that
red is not a good color for her is not the truth; it's your opinion. Sharing
your thoughts or ideas about the best course of action is not the truth, it's
your opinion. Someone else may have a different, equally valid point of
view. The truth tool is different because it goes right to the heart of your
experience. Your truth is the story you tell yourself, and the ways in which
you share it with others.

The best way to think about telling your truth is to imagine you
are giving an *internal weather report*. Based on the principles of conscious
living taught by Drs. Gay and Kathlyn Hendricks, an internal weather report means you are telling the truth about your internal experience. Take a

your fourth power tool is: tell the truth

moment right now and try your truth on for size. First off, look around you. What do you **notice?** If you could objectively describe what is around you, what would you say? Now, take a breath and **check in with your body,** scan it from head to toe, and notice what's going on inside you. Is there tightness between your shoulder blades, a slight ache in the back of your head, or do you have a warm, relaxed feeling in the center of your body?

What **feeling** are you experiencing at this moment? A sense of contentment, some sadness, or a bit of anxiety? What is the story you are telling yourself right now; what are you **imagining,** what **assumptions** are you making, or how are you **interpreting** what you've just read? Right now, **how would you like things to be;** in short, what are your yearnings, desires, or goals?

The answers to these questions are *your* truth. Your truth comes from your heart and is your inner experience. As the Hendricks' explain in their book, *At the Speed of Life,* no one can argue with it, because it belongs to you. Your truth is not absolute—but it is what is true for you. Becoming aware of your own truth allows you to set healthy boundaries and make conscious choices. Communicating your truth with others puts it out in the open and creates a situation where a dialog can begin.

The Truth About You

The focus of your truth is two-fold: the truth you tell yourself, and the truth you share with others. When you tell yourself the truth, it is important to be completely forthright, *wholly* honest. You need to become conscious of all the things you would say aloud, as well as all the things you would like to leave unsaid. You need to pay attention to what you think, as well as those thoughts you try to deny because they make you uncomfortable. For example, don't leave pieces out just because you don't like the message they carry or because they don't match with the way you'd like to see yourself. That squirrelly feeling you get in your stomach every time you think about having lunch with your pregnant best friend tells you that the issue needs your attention—your honest and candid attention.

So how do you discern your truth in the midst of all the thoughts buzzing around in your head? How do you know if you are dodging something important, and telling yourself you're fine, when in fact, you're not? Again, take a moment to check the barometer of your internal experience. Ask yourself: *am I avoiding an issue because I don't want to deal with how I feel? Or, am I avoiding my own needs and feelings in a relationship because it seems easier right now than bringing up my thoughts? The key issue again is, what are you pretending not to know?*

From time to time, everyone avoids the truth with others and with themselves. Nonetheless, those things you pretend not to know stand between you and the opportunity to be happier and more comfortable with yourself, with other people, and with the events of your life. When you avoid the truth or pretend not to know certain things, you thwart your own prospects for growth and personal breakthrough.

You cannot move forward making conscious choices or setting healthy boundaries unless you take ownership in all aspects of your life. You cannot be in an honest exchange with someone else until you first get honest with yourself. Stepping into this kind of ownership starts when you tell *your* truth, first to yourself, and then to the people with whom you interact. Begin by acknowledging your world for how you really see it, and deal with it by keeping the dialogue in your own head authentic and accurate about your experiences.

The Truth About Your World

Some people face life as if they will wake up tomorrow and their problems will have miraculously gone away. They accumulate debt by living a lifestyle they cannot afford, always hoping that tomorrow will bring a financial windfall to get them out of their situation. They tell themselves, tomorrow their boss will be nicer, their spouse will stop drinking, or the stress in their lives will miraculously disappear. This is "pretending not to know" in its simplest form. It is dangerous because while you are pretending, you miss genuine opportunities to improve the situation as it really is. The truth is, it is impossible to heal something you do not first acknowledge. Seeing a situation as it is, and telling the truth about it, is a critical step to change, to healing, and to growth.

Miracles do happen. Likewise, a positive attitude helps you get through many situations and is always beneficial to you. But lying to yourself and telling yourself something isn't what it truly is only adds to your pain, frustration, and disappointment.

If you are reading this book, infertility is already a part of your world. You may or may not conceive a child one day, but if you put your life on hold, waiting for your miracle to happen, it means that, in truth, you really aren't living your life at all. And if you spend each day expecting someone or some thing to rescue you or change your reality, you are going to be disappointed and unhappy in every single tomorrow that comes, while missing other things that can actually give meaning to your life. No doctor, diet, herbs, or incantations can rescue you from this.

The World's Untruths

According to the national infertility association known as RESOLVE, infertility affects approximately ten percent of the US population, or more than seven million women of childbearing age.[6] Yet despite the fact that over two million American women annually seek medical assistance for issues of fertility, the vast majority of women worldwide face this problem alone.

Why?

For starters, it is hard, even for medical professionals, to agree upon a definition for infertility. How long does a woman

> *we teach others how to treat us by what we communicate to them, but most importantly, by how we treat ourselves*

try; how hard does she try without conceiving, before the world agrees she is dealing with infertility? When in the process of trying does it stop being called, "trying" and start being called, "failing"? Then there is the matter of primary infertility, meaning difficulty conceiving your first pregnancy, and secondary infertility, which occurs in women who give birth to one or more children but have difficulty achieving the second, third, or even subsequent pregnancy.

How can you be honest with yourself about a problem and the feelings it evokes when the problem itself is so difficult to define?

Infertility, by its very nature, is hard to characterize. Many standard medical textbooks define infertility as *failure to conceive after one year of unprotected sexual intercourse.* In recent years, this definition often is expanded to include the caveat: *failure to conceive after one year of unprotected sexual intercourse in women under the age of thirty-five or six months of unprotected sexual intercourse in women over the age of thirty-five.*

The effort to measure infertility in terms of the calendar has come about in large part as a way to establish a usable definition for health insurance

---

[6] RESOLVE. The National Infertility Association. See website http://www.resolve.org/

companies, which in itself is ironic considering how infrequently insurance companies cover the cost of infertility treatments. Telling yourself the truth about infertility, and the feelings it evokes, wouldn't be so difficult if only the whole issue had less gray area.

The World Health Organization estimates that more than eighty million people worldwide experience some form of infertility.[7] But the media communicates a story with a very different message. All those gorgeous television and movie star icons, (you know who they are) make delaying motherhood look like every woman's choice. When the media spotlights these beautiful women, young beyond their actual years, with their adorable offspring in tow, no one mentions that their pregnancies are often the result of years of stressful treatments and hundreds of thousands of dollars in cost.

Women in almost all countries are marrying at a later age and delaying motherhood longer. Thanks to increased focus on exercise, self-care, and sometimes cosmetic surgical procedures, many women at thirty-five now look and perhaps feel twenty-five; women of forty-five look and feel thirty-five. Women have become very skillful at holding on to their youth and the positive side effect is that they are using this extended youth as a time to focus on careers, travel, educations, and in general spend more time getting to know themselves and their spouse.

All of these things are wonderful except for the fact that no amount of exercise, health food, yoga, or Botox, stops or even slows the aging of the oocytes (eggs) within your ovaries. Unlike your partner, who produces sperm throughout adulthood, you are born with a fixed number of eggs that is never replenished or rejuvenated during your lifetime.

Most importantly, women know their biological clocks are ticking, but

---

[7] See website for the World Health Organization: http://www.who.int/reproductive-health/infertility/index.htm

few have any idea just how fast. In a study conducted in conjunction with the American Fertility Association,[8] over 12,000 women answered a fifteen-question survey on basic fertility facts. Of the group, only one woman answered every single question correctly—*that is one single woman out of 12,000-plus who knew with one-hundred percent accuracy the real truths about her own fertility!* Eighty-eight percent of the women who took the survey overestimated by five to ten years the age at which fertility begins to diminish. The cold, hard fact is that the overwhelming majority of women did not know that their capability to conceive a child begins to diminish while they are still in their twenties.

While the intent has not deliberately been to misinform, popular culture leads most women to believe things about fertility that simply are not the truth. If you learned, in the most painful of ways, that your life choices have now placed you in a situation where pregnancy is difficult, if not impossible, then you are angry. You justifiably feel anger at yourself for not knowing better and anger at all those forty-year old movie stars pushing designer baby carriages, as if it is the easiest thing in the world to do. Sadly, the real truths about fertility not only have the power to sneak up on you, but are as devastating as anything you will ever face.

Tell Yourself the Truth

While avoiding the reality of your world may lead you to stick your head in the sand and pretend your life is different than it really is, oddly enough, most women find it easy to pull their heads up just long enough to unleash a stream of cruel self-criticism. When you're struggling to conceive, you may, without realizing it, treat yourself pretty harshly. Misplaced shame and guilt can translate into some very negative (and untrue) self-talk. Until

[8] See website for the American Fertility Association: http://www.theafa.org/faqs/afa_whatmotherdidnotsay.html

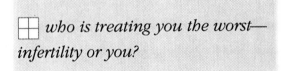 *who is treating you the worst— infertility or you?*

you can move past the anger you may feel over being **deceived** about the true facts of fertility, it can be very hard not to beat yourself up about your situation.

Think about the things you routinely tell yourself and then sit down with paper and pen. Listen to your own self-talk and make a list of the comments you make to yourself. Your list will be quite revealing.

One of Marina's clients, who had been struggling with infertility for a number of months, admitted she constantly felt angry with herself. When she sat down and performed this exercise, she was shocked by what she discovered. Listening in on her self-talk, she found herself saying things like, "Forget it, I'm just a waste. I can't have a baby. I can't do anything."

When she genuinely paid attention to what she was saying to herself, she could easily see the impact her critical, self-punishing attitude was having on her stress and the feeling of self-defeat with which she was struggling. Imagine trying to excel at a sport if all you ever heard was negative talk. Think about trying to advance in your job if you only receive criticism from others. Envision trying to do *anything* well if positive reinforcement is missing and all you hear is an off-putting and pessimistic report on your failings.

Negative self-talk is not only detrimental, it is *a lie!* When you tell yourself you are a failure because you cannot conceive a child, you are not telling the truth.

Sometimes it is easier to understand a situation in your own life if you frame it in the context of something similar but different. For example, an elderly gentleman experienced a painful life crisis on top of a life crisis when shortly after his wife of fifty years received a diagnosis of Alzheimer's disease, he was diagnosed with a serious form of skin cancer.

Because you are standing outside his life, you can clearly see that this man was not responsible for either of these catastrophic events. Yet he directed much of his hurt and his anger at himself.

He saw his body as failing him at the time he most needed to be there for his wife. He struggled with thoughts that, if he had only used sunscreen years ago, or spent less time on the golf course, maybe he would not have had this cancer today. Of course, when this man was younger, no one talked about the relationship between sun exposure and skin cancer. He couldn't have known to diligently use sunscreen in 1952, because at that time, no one was aware that a suntan was anything other than healthy looking.

Obviously, if he had less exposure to the sun and had played golf less often, he might have lowered his odds of getting skin cancer. However, without the beneficial exercise and relaxation he gained from playing golf, he might also have died from a heart attack many years earlier. If his loving wife had been able to communicate with him, she would have been the first person to tell him that she did not hold him accountable for any of the problems they faced.

You can see all these things clearly, while this man, distraught with his grief, did not. Daily he told himself he had failed his wife. At a time when he should have been focusing on his own health in order to get through the cancer treatments that lay ahead of him, he was focused instead on his anger and frustration with himself.

But how different is this seventy-four year old gentlemen from you or from many women who are faced with fertility challenges?

Chapter 3 reminded you that you would not be angry and say negative things to another woman just because she was struggling to conceive a child. So why make yourself feel bad by saying negative things *about you,* to you? Who is treating you the worst—infertility or you?

The ideas you developed about self-blame, misplaced responsibility, or how things are going to be miraculously different when you get up in the morning are not truths. They are simply concepts you've invented based on your assumptions, past experiences, or unrealistic expectations about yourself or the situation. Many times women fall short of being who they think they should be because they have created an image of a woman no one can live up to. Living your truth begins with taking a step toward yourself and making the effort to examine both the truths and the lies you tell yourself. Look at your face in the mirror and ask yourself again, "What am I pretending not to know?"

Retelling Your Story

While it is not always easy to change your thoughts, consider that much of your self-talk is simply a habit you have fallen into because you have done it so often it seems natural. If you have always been self-critical, then this approach to life has become your pattern. But habits are only comfortable because you have done them frequently. Cross your arms in front of you by folding them across your chest. Look to see which arm is on top when you fold your arms in this way. Now, cross them again, this time deliberately putting your other arm on top.

Changing the pattern of which arm you put on top of the other will feel uncomfortable. You may even have to look at your arms in order consciously to cross your arms in the opposite way from which you usually do it. But there is no right or wrong way to cross your arms. The way you typically do it merely feels right and is the easiest to do because it is the way you typically do it. If you make a conscious effort to change the way you cross

> *changing how you talk to yourself takes the same type of deliberate effort that you need to break any habit*

your arms for the next thirty or forty times you do it, the new way would eventually come to feel more natural than the old way.

Changing how you talk to yourself takes the same type of deliberate effort that you need to change or break any habit. One of the best techniques to help you do this is to take a step back from your own situation and reframe your story. For example, when you read the story of the seventy-four year old gentlemen, you were on the outside looking in on his life. That perspective allowed you to be objective, and in so doing, you gained clarity, and had compassion for his plight. You realized when he made choices in the past, he was doing the best he could with the information he had at that time, and that he was not responsible for his illness.

You can use this same strategy when you are distraught, or facing a stressful situation. Simply step back, and turn your story into someone else's story. Like a playwright, write down what you are struggling with in your life, but cast an imaginary character in your own role. Give her a name, and become a spectator of her situation. Write down what happens in imaginary Maria, Loretta, or Olivia's life. Describe how she feels, what her conflicts are, and the thoughts that are going through her head. You can gain amazing clarity about your most personal issues when you step back and view your own life from an outside point of view.

Once you have identified your character's dilemma, bear in mind that as the playwright or author of this script, you have only one obligation: to keep your main character's life on target. When she faces painful or unpleasant experiences, think through the best choices for her to make, the most rational, the most beneficial. Write out what she will say to others and how she will act when she makes that choice. Allow your journal to become a way to separate your old negative habits from those you are now consciously creating, choices that are empowering and honest.

Your leading lady is human—not perfect, indestructible, or a superhero. Have compassion for her shortcomings and struggles, and work to steer her clear of choices that are hurtful or self-destructive. Be mindful of the tools of making conscious choices, taking healthy responsibility, and telling the truth, as she explores how to create a life of balance—honoring herself, while being there for others. Along the way, she will stumble, she will make mistakes, but your job is to keep picking her up, with love and compassion, and to keep reminding her that every fall provides another chance to grow, to regroup and move forward.

As you use journaling and scriptwriting to help bring perspective to your experiences, you are giving yourself a gift. You are allowing yourself the opportunity to step back and see clearly in someone else's life what patterns and which old habits may be blocking you in your own life.

The bonus is that changing your life's story allows you to focus on the truth about the *whole* of who you are. Changing your life's story enables you to connect with the fact that you are not your infertility—it is just a medical condition that is happening to you. Who you are is a loving daughter and wife, a committed volunteer, a loyal friend. This is the truth of the whole of you.

Truth Talk With Your Spouse or Partner

Make a very deliberate choice to start telling the truth to your partner. Take the risk to say the tough stuff, the thoughts that get you thinking, "Oh, I could never tell him that." If you find yourself holding back from communicating what is true for you because you imagine it will evoke an emotionally charged response, look out! This is the bright red flag signaling, *this is the very thing you need to be talking about.*

Diane and David experienced firsthand the impact of this communication obstacle. After many months of unsuccessful fertility treatment and growing tension in their relationship, they decided they needed couples counseling. The strain of medical treatment was taking its toll on Diane, and she felt physically and emotionally exhausted. While she needed time to regroup before she could consider their next step, David was solely focused on the next treatment option.

Rather than talking about her need to take a break, Diane kept silent. Wracked with guilt at being unable to conceive, she complied with her husband's expectations and continued through phase after phase of treatment. Underneath this silence however, a growing hostility was brewing; it was only a matter of time before Diane reached her breaking point.

What had really happened here?

Rather than taking care of herself and communicating about her needs and feelings, Diane had abandoned herself. The very things she needed to talk about—her need to take a break, her fear of disappointing her husband, her own feelings of guilt and unworthiness—she avoided because she feared an emotional reaction from her husband. In doing so, she was being dishonest—she was pretending things were fine, when in fact she was suffering. And she was making some dangerous assumptions about David, which she followed by keeping silent and acting as if these assumptions were true. Unfortunately, Diane was making choices that were grossly unfair to herself, to David, and to the relationship!

In order for this relationship to come back into a place of balance,

⊞ if you want to know what you really believe, look at your life

the couple needed to address both the issue of responsibility and of communication. When Diane imagined David would not be able to handle what she had to say, she was taking too much responsibility for him and not enough for herself. In an effort to protect him for what she suspected to be the harsh truth of her feelings, their relationship suffered. Diane felt distanced from her husband, and she harbored both anger and resentment toward him and herself. Not until she was ready to take responsibility solely for her own feelings, and tell her husband the truth as she experienced it, were they able to move toward healing their relationship and making decisions that worked for both of them.

This pattern of taking too much responsibility for someone you care about and not enough for yourself is a very common one for many women. The idea of disappointing someone you care about can make you so uncomfortable that there is the temptation to go along with what the other person wants (or what you think he or she wants) in order to avoid discomfort. In reality, this behavior is just another form of control—trying to control the situation, the response of the other person, and the ultimate outcome. The giving you are doing is not authentic; it is not clean. Rather, it comes under the heading of "giving with an agenda".

Control issues can crop up in many different ways during fertility challenges. People want to, and expect to, control their bodies. The frustration athletes feel when they cannot propel their body to perform at a higher level is partly because people feel if they do certain things, i.e., train, exercise, prepare for their sport, then they should be entitled to see certain responses or benefits from their actions. As people age, they feel angry when their bodies betray them. They cannot see as well as they once did and their mobility diminishes with time. Controlling one's own body feels as if it should be an entitlement, but fertility challenges slap you smack in the face with the fact that, *in truth,* some things about your body *are completely outside of your control.* You can make every positive lifestyle choice you can imagine, and still, *it is what it is.*

When Diane was able to give up control of how she wanted David to see her, and simply said to her husband, "I need a break, but I'm afraid to tell you because I imagine I'll be disappointing you," the logjam broke. They were finally able to talk about their fears and hopes together. Their honesty with each other created the intimacy necessary to grow closer as a couple.

As you permit your husband to love you for who you are, not for who *you think* he wants you to be, you open your marriage to receive another one of the gifts of infertility. Many studies[9] have found that couples who struggle with fertility are actually closer and have better communication than couples who sail through life without such challenges. Your shared experience with infertility forces you to deal with tough issues that a lot of other people have not yet faced, or may never have to face.

Weathering the infertility storm together means you and your husband or partner need to develop communication proficiencies and coping skills that are up to the challenge you face. The good news is not only are these the skills that affect your situation now, they also carry over into other aspects of your life and your marriage. Rather than believing you need to project an image to be loved, you will know what it feels like to love, and be loved for your authentic self.

---

[9] Domar, Alice D., and Kelly, Alice Lesch. *Conquering Infertility: Dr. Alice Domar's Mind/Body Guide to Enhancing Fertility and Coping with Infertility.* New York: Penguin Group, 2002, p. 17.

Building on the Truth

The truths that accompany fertility have a subtle (and not so subtle) way of becoming all-consuming, creeping into every aspect of a marriage. However, there are ways to give infertility the attention it merits, without letting it overwhelm your relationship with your spouse. Yes, fertility issues are important, but it is equally as important to keep them in their place.

One easy solution is to put aside a preset amount of time each day of anywhere from ten to twenty minutes for talking together about your most current feelings on the subject. The amount of time you set aside depends on how you are feeling, what issues you are dealing with, and even how long you've been in treatment. Don't think that it's corny or contrived to set a timer so each of you gets equal talking time. Setting a timer allows you to tweak the balance, especially if one of you tends to be the "over talker" and the other more the listener. Make sure each of you gets to talk without interruption, and then you can switch. You may even want to take turns each night going first. Keep in mind there are certain times when you definitely do not want to plan to talk, like before bed, when you're running out of the house in the morning, or any other occasion when you feel pressed for time.

In communicating, be careful not to belabor or repeat the same points over and over. Say what you need to say, and then listen—*really listen*—to your spouse. Give your partner only good information, meaning tell him the truth the way it really is for you, not the way you think you should feel, or the way you think he expects you to feel. This strategy allows each partner to feel listened to and stay involved. The bonus is that you will be able to spend the rest of your time together enjoying each other, pursuing other interests, and NOT focusing on the topic of infertility.

Truth Talk With Your World

The same types of truth-telling strategies essential in your marriage also need to extend beyond the bounds of your marriage into your relationships with other people. Don't make the assumption that your friends, your boss, or your mother can read your mind and know what you need. It is your responsibility to let others know what you want and what works for you. Just like you would tell your husband that you want him to accompany you to a doctor's appointment, you can make the same request of a close friend. If your family seems clueless about your fertility treatments, and you want them to be informed, then teach them. Give them helpful magazine articles and direct them to websites. If you want certain people to call and check on you after a doctor's appointment, tell them. If your best friend calls too much, tactfully let her know this too.

Telling your truth is the path to self-discovery and authentic relationships. It is the vehicle that facilitates *many times women fall short of being who they think they should be because they have created an image of a woman that no one can live up to* taking healthy responsibility for your needs, actions, and choices, while letting go of what does not belong to you and what no longer serves you. The idea that "we teach others how to treat us," comes alive when you tell your truth. You are communicating to your world, "I am worth it!" Your self-validation creates the model for others to follow. Your relationships with yourself and others become vital, dynamic, and free!

FROM MARINA'S CASE FILES ON
Danielle R.

Oftentimes, the very life skills that, allow us as children, to get through some tough situations within our families, are the very ones that stand in the way of our developing healthy relationships as adults. This was certainly the case with Danielle, who, as the only daughter of an abusive, alcoholic father, learned well the childhood admonition that it's better "to be seen and not heard." From there, it was only a short step to believing that stoicism was synonymous with strength.

Danielle was a late starter in the baby game. As she describes it, she spent her time working hard at her family's business, "but snoozing through her biological alarm clock." To her surprise, an unplanned pregnancy, and its resulting miscarriage at almost forty-one years old, woke her up to her deep desire to have a baby. But baby making is a tricky thing, and not always responsive to even one's best efforts. So two years, and numerous fertility tests and procedures later, Danielle was still childless.

Danielle is a woman who was accustomed to success. As she learned in childhood, the formula for getting the job done had been to keep her head down and her feelings in check. But the parameters of this situation conformed to none of these old rules, and she found herself overwhelmed at the enormity of her grief. Unfortunately, Danielle had created a life where she literally had nowhere to turn. She described her husband as logical and somewhat detached, and she feared that if she allowed him to see the depth of her despair, he would emotionally abandon her in much the same way her father had. She had even honed this implacable persona outside her home as well. Her private life was strictly kept out of her associations with work colleagues, and even within her small circle of friends, she was seen as the one who "had it all together."

As time went on, and the pressure continued to build, Danielle's personal life began to disassemble. There were outbursts of anger at her husband, isolation from her friends, reprimands for her distractedness at work. It was in the midst of this personal chaos that Danielle decided to reach out and seek counseling. Although Danielle didn't realize it, the self-protective persona that had gotten her through her childhood and up to this point in her life, was cracking. She needed to learn to acknowledge her feelings, and reach out for support.

Fortunately for Danielle, she showed the same commitment to this process as she did to every other area of her life. In a sense, she started the process of introducing herself to herself, and listened, perhaps for the first time, to the truth of her feelings, her experiences, her needs, and her desires. As her sense of internal awareness grew, she took the next step, and began to tell her truth to her husband, and even to a few close friends. She began to attend an infertility support group, and saw her own struggles and longing mirrored in the women there. Yes, there were stops and starts along the way, a marriage that needed mending, and friendships that were lost, while others were gained. However, along the way, Danielle learned that the true meaning of strength was not stoicism, as she had once believed, but the vulnerability that allowed her to honor her truth.

This lesson would serve her well as she continued on her journey to parenthood. Unable to become pregnant, she and her husband finally came to the question of whether to use donor eggs. At first, this was difficult for Danielle. She felt guilt for having waited so long, and shame, for not being able to do something that was supposed to be natural. She also had concerns about whether she would be able to bond with a child who would be biologically unrelated to her. But Danielle had learned to confront and talk through her feelings, and as a result, these doubts held no power over her. When she finally made the decision to move forward, it was from a place of peace and of resolution.

This made the welcoming of her baby girl truly a celebration.

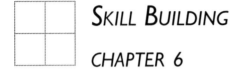

SKILL BUILDING

CHAPTER 6

1. Often such sentences begin with:

    Select someone, such as your husband or a good friend, and share with him or her the things you have learned about telling *your truth*. Then enlist your partner's help to practice telling your truth. For example, take turns and each of you share with the other simple statements that express what is true for you. Your statements will be brief; typically something you can deliver in one breath, and will represent your personal weather report. Often such sentences begin with:

    I feel...   I notice...   or I'm imagining...

    For example: I feel excited; I notice I have butterflies in my stomach; I'm imagining you're getting upset.

    The first person who veers off, and shares an opinion or a concept instead of a personal truth is out!

    After sharing your weather report, consider whether sharing your truth was easier or harder than you expected?

2. Danielle R. (in the case study for Chapter 6) provides a powerful example of how, during childhood, you often learn to hide the truth of who you are and what you feel, in order to cope with difficult situations. Unfortunately, too often, rather than dealing with the truth of what's really going on, children learn to judge or criticize themselves. To take a step into the impact of this, take your journal and list negative, self-critical things you have told yourself at least three times during your life. Now close your eyes and imagine that you are sitting across from your five-year-old self and saying these things, three times each to the little girl you used to be. Take a breath and notice how you feel. Now ask yourself: what do I want her to believe is the truth?

3. Once negative self-talk gets going, it can feel like a runaway train. The

following exercise called *TLC*, (**T**ruth **L**ies **C**reate) is adapted from *Focus Seminars of Kansas City*. This particular exercise is a great way to separate the truth from the lies you tell yourself, and get that train of yours back on the right track.

The next time you find yourself in a spiral of negative self-talk, pull out your journal and write verbatim what you hear yourself saying. Next, mark through every statement that is not working for you, that does not serve your highest good, and that does not reflect the best of who you are (the lies). Leave the rest (the truth) on your page.

Danielle's willingness to do this exercise was critical in her gaining self-awareness and helped her clarify her next step. Here's an excerpt from her process:

> "No matter how hard I try, I can't seem to make this happen. I am such a failure! I can see why my husband does not want to talk to me. How could he love me when I can't even give him a child? I feel lost and so confused. No one understands me. I am tired of having to deal with all of this alone. I wish I could find someone to talk to. I am tired of hurting."

After Danielle crossed out the lies, she realized how she was beating herself up and creating a no-win situation.

> "No matter how hard I try, I can't seem to make this happen. ~~I am such a failure! I can see why my husband does not want to talk to me. How could he love me when I can't even give him a child?~~ I feel lost and so confused. ~~No one understands me.~~ I am tired of having to deal with all of this alone. I wish I could find someone to talk to. I am tired of hurting."

The words Danielle was left with was her truth; no one could argue with these words. This truth allowed her to acknowledge her need for counseling.

4. Try this yourself and then read the lies you have told yourself. What kind
    of impact do you think that negative self-talk has on you? How do you think
    they hold you back?

    Finally, read the truth—what works—in the way you speak to yourself. Make
    a list of these statements, changing words as needed to language that will
    empower you. Read your list aloud. Decide what you want to create in your
    life by embracing your new self-talk.

Your Fifth Power Tool: Take Quiet Space

Do you remember when you could pull a blanket over your head and become invisible? As a child, you saw the value in empty packing crates, tents made by draping a sheet over two chairs, and even just the dark and sometimes dusty space underneath your bed.

You sought quiet nooks and hidden places. No matter how much you loved your family and your friends, you also cherished time in your special place to cry, laugh, sort through your feelings, daydream, and pretend, all in blissful privacy.

But little girls grow up. Sitting underneath the stairs or on the big branch of the maple tree is replaced by tiny dormitory rooms or apartments shared with housemates or a new boyfriend. You move further and further away from the little girl who instinctively understood she needed her own special place, even if it was only a corner, even if it was only for a little while.

Many people come home from busy, conversation-filled days at their

| □ *your fifth power tool is: take quiet space* |

place of business, only to turn on the television the minute they hit the door of their quietly waiting home. Busy women often find that when unexpected free time crops up in their schedule, they call a friend or make a plan to fill the time and space with another activity and another person. Like the old video game of Pac-Man, engaging with someone or something becomes a way to gobble up every corner of empty space in your life. Little by little, you move away from being the child who loved hiding places to being an adult who literally has no place to hide. The more time you spend with others, the easier it becomes to overlook the need for alone time with yourself.

Creating Time and Creating a Space

Why is it so important for you to structure quiet time into your day?

The answer to this question has a lot to do with the modern demands of daily life. Gone are the days of prior generations when extended periods of quiet time were woven into the natural fabric of living. Once, whole lives were lived within walking distance, and chores and responsibilities, indoors or outside, were often done in quiet, in sync with a slower rhythm of life.

No more. Today, life is busy and compressed. When you squeeze in a 7:30 A.M. doctor's appointment, with the hope that afterwards you can rush to work on time, there is no opportunity to process the good or bad news you just received. You stuff your feelings and sideline your thoughts because you have to return to an office full of people, a classroom of children, or other similarly demanding situation. But when is your time to sort it all out?

The hectic pace of modern life makes it essential that you *consciously choose* to take quiet space. People need private time; they need a measure of quietude each day to counterbalance the busyness, noise, and overload of people that fills their waking hours. This need is present on a day-to-day basis, when nothing special is going on. Throw in fertility struggles, and the need is raised a thousand fold. With the barrage of information hitting you daily, the number of things you have to juggle, and the important decisions you need to make, (especially if you're undergoing fertility treatment) quiet time is your critical space for sorting it all out. Yes, you need support from others. But, as you've already realized, discerning your own feelings is not always easy. Plus, there are simply some decisions and some choices you can only resolve in the quiet of your own heart. Creating a private special place—a physical place that is all your own—is a way to give yourself the time and space you critically need.

A Place All Your Own

When you spend time in your special place, you are, in a sense, taking off the face you wear for the rest of the world. Like washing off your make-up and changing from a business suit and heels to your favorite sweatpants and t-shirt, going to your "place" lets you be comfortably you.

Whether your home is large or small, try to find a place that can become your personal space. This may be a room or it may be only a favorite chair tucked away in a corner. As long as you can make it feel like yours and yours alone, even a very tiny space will work. If you cannot easily figure out where your special place should be, try enlisting the assistance of your spouse or partner. Put your heads together and re-think the way the two of you use your home so that you can carve out a place just for you.

As you create your space, think back to the places that attracted you when you were a child. Did you like them best because no one else could see you there? Was the attraction that your special place was small and just the right size for you, or perhaps you liked it because from your space, you could see treetops and a beautiful view? Think of ways to incorporate the same types of things that drew you to your childhood secret place into your new, grown-up, special place. Be sure to include items that feel good to you and bring you comfort. Perhaps you appreciate a snuggly pillow, fresh flowers, a scented candle, an elegant notebook, or your favorite pen. Pick items that indulge your senses and soothe your soul.

The space you create is yours to use each day. Put aside time when you will not be disturbed, even ten, twenty, or thirty minutes. Give yourself the same respect you give to others. When your best friend calls and says, "I need to talk," you set aside time to spend with her and listen to her express her thoughts. When your spouse or partner says, "Honey, let's discuss this," you quickly respond to his request. Do the same thing for yourself, and as you do, you will notice that something amazing happens. You will begin to associate your space with the solace and quietude you are investing there. After a while, just sinking into your special chair will trigger a sense of letting go, in your body, and in your mind. Your space will be a place for you to come home to yourself—to think, to reflect, regroup, and to process your feelings and experiences.

Coming Into Your Own

How you use your quiet space is very personal. You've tried on enough clothing labeled "one size fits all" to know that someone else's idea of what will work for you may be way off base. Fertility challenges are intimate experiences. Causes, cures, and coping mechanisms, can be unique and totally distinctive from one woman to another, and even totally different for you from one stage in your journey to another. While the seven tools taught in this book are universal, how you use them, personalize them, and take them to the next level, is all about finding what works best for you at this moment.

Journaling, meditation, visualization, and self-questioning are all effective devices to use in your quiet space to help you gain peace, clarity, and self-understanding. As you read more about each technique, look not only for ways that you know will be comfortable for you, but also be open to trying unexpected methods you have never considered a "fit" for you. Be open to learning and experimenting with new things. Like trying on that dress that doesn't "look like your usual style" sometimes, stepping out of your comfort zone introduces new and powerfully effective elements into your life that you would have never thought were right for you.

Often times, a small ritual of some sort can be very helpful in allowing you to make the transition from the outer world of the rest of your life, into the inner world of just you. Experiment until you find a process that works for you and can become consistent. Although one size never fits all, you may be surprised to find a perfect fit in a way you never expected to find it. For example, while the idea of creating a symbolic guide to talk to and to lead you into your quiet space may sound too "new age" for you, remember that your childhood imaginary friend was an excellent confidante and sounding board. Envisioning a wise and nurturing *nonna*, a gentle doe with finely tuned animal instincts and strong survival skills, or a protective guardian angel are all excellent devices to call on if doing so helps you shift from a noisy, busy world to a hushed and meditative place.

A different but equally valid approach to help you transition into your quiet space could come in the form of lighting a candle or brewing a cup of tea. While food itself should not be one of the comfort tools you call on in your quiet space, the act of brewing tea is recognized across many cultures for its ceremonial and ritualistic value. Waiting for the water to boil, watching the steam curl above your favorite lapis-blue china cup, the incense-like aroma of the chamomile, and even the gentle tinkling sound of your spoon as it swirls the tea in small circles, can all become markers your brain will come to recognize as part of your personal routine for stepping into a time of reflection. Arriving at your place of mental quiet is a learned skill. Repetition of your transition routine serves as a signal to your body and your mind that now is the time to slow down and to unwind.

There is a myth that teaches people that all the answers they ever need are found within themselves. In fact, the accurate version of this wisdom is that within one's self is everything she will ever need *to discover* the answers. Right now, the reason that you don't feel as if you have all the answers (or perhaps any of the answers) about what is going on in your life is because you really don't. Just because a problem is yours and yours alone does not mean that the resolution is also found contained within your conscious mind. Here's a startling newsflash: the part of your brain that figures things out is about the size of a quarter! That's pretty limited when you consider that you have at your disposal a universe of possibilities when it comes to answering questions. In other words, where you "travel" when you are in your quiet space may be to your own consciousness; it may be to your own subconscious; or it may be to a type of wisdom that flows, not from the inside out, but from the greater universe into your heart and your mind. Go to your quiet place and listen. As a Buddhist proverb says, "When the student is ready, the teacher will appear."

Making It Write

You may discover that now is an ideal time to take your notebook and use it to express whatever comes to the surface…your thoughts, feelings, hopes, and fears. The journal writing process is very powerful: it's almost as if writing the words on paper gives your thoughts validity and substance.

Some people enjoy the cathartic and creative process of writing. Other people view it like a nagging homework assignment. The only way you will know if writing is an effective way for you to gain greater self-awareness is to try it, welcoming the possibility that you will find journaling to be a beneficial and useful part of how you utilize your quiet space.

Language can focus your feelings in a way that no other process does. Sometimes when you use a journal to help you understand yourself better, you will find yourself writing in a very premeditated way. You may move through your words slowly and purposefully. Other times, the act of writing seems to flow like a river, one word spilling into the next, each with a life of its own. While these experiences are very different from each other, each is an enlightening, beneficial, and often, cathartic process.

Poetry is another form of writing that can powerfully channel your experience. Within the context of journaling, poetry can be loosely written, taking whatever form you want it to take. You need not be a poet to enjoy writing in this way and your words may not even resemble a traditional poem. Poetic writing however, can allow you to express feelings or relate memories that include specific details, such as sights, sounds, and smells.

When you write, you take your story from ideas and concepts to actual language. This language helps you to translate that vague sense into something concrete. People often say that after a dream, if they tell the details of their dream to someone else immediately upon awakening, they are better able to recall the dream later. This happens because they took something (the dream) that came out of their subconscious mind and converted it to the very conscious-mind concepts of words, phrases, and sentences.

Keep in mind as you write, your words are for no one's eyes but yours.

Your journal is a place for your innermost thoughts, so the manner in which you write is also personal—whether it is big, angry, bold blocks of letters, or sentences that run together without any semblance of punctuation or grammar. Let this writing follow your stream of consciousness, and let it flow out of you and onto the page. Sometimes you may choose to direct your writing toward someone else, like open dialogues (or rants) written to your spouse or partner, the child you have not conceived, your doctor, your mother, or even a symbol that holds spiritual or religious meaning for you. Your written words may become prayers, letters to yourself as a child, or letters to your future self. Or your writing may not have any recognizable form at all. Don't force your writing to become anything preconceived. Let insights flow in either direction, with your only goal being to recognize new perceptions as they reveal themselves.

When psychotherapist Ira Progoff returned to civilian life after serving in the US Army during World War II, he found himself struggling to reconcile the horrors of war and how precariously close he felt society came to destroying itself during Hitler's reign. Progoff was particularly disturbed by the Nazi book burning of the 1930's, and how he feared such incidents raised the possibility of all documented insights of the ages somehow being destroyed. However, through his research on journaling, Progoff was able to put these fears to rest. In his book, *The Practice of Process Meditation*, Progoff explains that if such a thing were to happen, the world would "simply draw new spiritual scriptures from the same source out of which the old ones came..." What Progoff is saying is that while *you* may not specifically have a type of wisdom within yourself, you still have access to it by making yourself open to understanding the wisdom existing within the universe.

The Progoff Intensive Journal® Program is a tool designed to help people use writing to access and understand both conscious and subconscious messages. From his workshops on journaling came his book, *At a Journal Workshop,* published in 1975. This book has been helpful to so many people that more than thirty years after it first came to print, it is still in publication. You may find this book useful to help you use journaling as a self-help, self-healing tool. As Progoff says of his studies into the individual's ability to recover from trauma or crisis, "…I became aware of how vast and self-replenishing are the resources of the human spirit."

The benefits of journal writing on emotional and physical wellbeing are also well documented in the book, *Mind-Body Harmony, How to Resist and Recover from Auto-Immune Diseases.* In this book, Dr. Terry Willard suggests that journaling is a great way to release the emotional baggage that is so easy to pick up on a day to day basis. This unprocessed "emotional roughage" has a detrimental effect on the body, he claims, with healthy people oftentimes developing the most difficult health issues. In fact, he noticed that many of these otherwise healthy patients studied, shared the common traits of being emotionally sensitive, and somewhat perfectionistic, a potential recipe, he says, for autoimmune issues. While the jury is still out on the link between immunity problems and fertility challenges, there is no debate over the fact that journaling can provide a valuable outlet for releasing the "worry, tension, stress, and emotional crisis" that have proven detrimental effects on the body.

Your Written Word

What you do with your journaling after you write it is up to you. Some people like to keep their journals as something to look back on—to help them recall where they were and measure how far they have come. Others find the memories too painful, and they would just as soon let them go. You could choose to have your writing bound into books you cherish; to shred it; or even to start a ritual where you ceremonially burn what you've written. The simple act of watching the smoke rise up from your charring, shriveling words can serve as a symbolic way to release and let go of what no longer serves you.

One of the interesting things about the smoke that you watch twist and swirl above your burning pages comes from another observation Ira Progoff documented in *At a Journal Workshop*. Progoff notes this insight from the ancient Chinese philosopher, Lao Tzu, "the growth principle in life, which he called the *Tao,* is too elusive to be named or to be grasped at all…personal growth is…like smoke going out the chimney. We know it exists, but its shape keeps changing."

The Art of Self-Expression

Expressing your feelings is not limited to the written word. Creating art is a powerful and personal way to give substance to your experience and it can be enormously helpful in identifying your feelings and healing your grief. Do not worry if you cannot so much as draw a straight line; all that is necessary is a willingness to explore and to heal.

Art materials can include unlined paper, colored pencils or crayons, poster board, scissors and glue for collages, oil pastels, or tempera paints, even photos or magazine images. You may want to gather some items for your artwork, and keep them with your journal in your personal space. Then, simply let your intuition guide you to express what is in your heart.

Meditation and Visualization

Much has been written about the benefits of visual imagery and meditation, and the ways they can facilitate relaxation, enhance personal growth, even speed recovery from illness. Research shows a definitive correlation between fertility and stress. A Harvard Medical School study published in the medical journal, *Fertility and Sterility*, in 2000, found that of 185 women who had been trying to conceive for at least one year, fifty-five percent of those who attended a mind/body program became pregnant within a year, in comparison to just twenty percent in the control group.

Invest the time to discover which stress-reduction skills work best for you. Visual imagery is an option that allows you to accompany your breathing with a scene that is particularly peaceful for you—perhaps walking along the shore of a beach, or a quiet, green meadow, ripe with flowers. When you practice imagery, be sure to use all your senses; feel the cool breeze on your face as you are walking on the shore of the ocean, smell the salty air, feel the stickiness of the salt on your skin, the softness of the wet sand on your feet. The purpose of this type of imagery is to help you leave your real-world tensions and mentally vacation for a while in a place of peace and restfulness.

If you want your quiet time to be about relaxing or unwinding, you can calm your mind by taking long, slow, deep breaths…into a count of four…and then out to a count of four. Repeating a word or phrase you find particularly calming, like "peace" or "all is well," on the exhale is also helpful in encouraging a relaxed state.

Westernizing the practice of meditation is largely due to the work of Herbert Benson, MD, of Harvard University. In his groundbreaking book, *The Relaxation Response*, Dr. Benson recommends four simple steps to elicit stress relief and relaxation. The following exercise is adapted from this book:

1. Find a quiet space and sit in a comfortable position.
2. Close your eyes and consciously relax your muscles. Feel yourself

   sitting in your chair. Feel your feet on the ground.

3. Become aware of your breathing. As you exhale, say a word, such as
    "one" silently to yourself. Breathe naturally.

4. Assume a passive attitude toward any intrusive thoughts, meaning
    that when they occur, say a mental "oh well" and let them go—
    don't resist them, but don't hold on to them either. A good way to
    imagine this is to think of every thought as a cloud: even if you try,
    you can't hold on to it, so just let it float away. Continue for ten to
    twenty minutes. Do this once or twice a day.

As effective as this method is, his follow-up research, published in, *Beyond the Relaxation Response,* emphasized what he calls the "faith factor." Benson discovered that the power of this technique rises exponentially when you choose a word or phrase that is consistent with your personal, spiritual belief system. In the words of Dr. Benson, "…a personally important word or phrase…can provide a greater calming effect on your mind than you might achieve with a neutral focus word."

For Christians, for example, Dr. Benson suggests a line from the Our Father or Lord's Prayer, such as "hallowed be thy name," or the word, "Shalom," for someone from a Jewish heritage. Muslims may want to use the word for God, "Allah," or for Hindus the passage, "Joy is inward," from the Bhagavad-Gita. The only limitation is that if you choose a phrase, rather than a word, it should be short enough to be said silently as you exhale. This type of meditation can be a very helpful way to access the power of your faith, especially if you are dealing with fertility struggles.

Alternative Methods: Putting Yourself Into the Equation

For Amanda, three years into her infertility treatments, visualizing that she was an integral part of her own fertility management also helped her move away from her feeling of helplessness. Amanda took her visualizations to another level by applying them in a way she be- *we can best give to others from a full cup* lieved increased her likelihood of conceiving. Using a specific visualization process described by authors Niravi B. Payne and Brenda Lane Richardson in the book, *The Whole Person Fertility Program,*^SM allowed Amanda the peace of mind that she had done absolutely everything possible to become pregnant. Payne and Richardson explain this particular visualization as being, "specifically designed to celebrate your fertility and to help prepare your endometrium, the mucous membrane lining of the uterus, to receive a fertilized egg and hold the pregnancy to term."

Amanda embraced this type of imagery. She found it both comforting and relaxing, and she felt empowered by an inner strength. Donna's story, however, was very different. Already a great believer in "mind over matter," Donna also jumped into visualization techniques soon after realizing that her pregnancy was not coming easily. Daily, Donna worked at visualizing her body preparing for pregnancy and ultimately nurturing a fertilized ovum. But a year later, when Donna was still not pregnant, such visualizations began to be a very touchy subject for her. Well-meaning friends would give her books on the power of mental imagery. Even strangers would somehow manage to tell her how their cousin's neighbor or their boss's daughter-in-law had conceived through self-hypnosis or by going to see a specialist in visualization and mind-body healing. Donna came to see herself as failing on two fronts.

Alternative methods have a very valid place in treating a range of mental and physical conditions. Holistic options, such as acupuncture, herbal medicine, and homeopathy may be the best choice for dealing with infertility issues. At other times, conventional medicine may offer a woman's only hope for conceiving. Whether treatments are conventional or alternative, the line that separates hope from desperation can sometimes become blurred.

When Donna failed to conceive, she was frustrated. After a year of visualization techniques to prepare her body for pregnancy, and still no pregnancy, Donna was not only frustrated, she was now angry with herself for somehow failing to visualize with sufficient faith or intensity to result in conception. When these types of body-preparation visualization techniques do not result in pregnancy, they can leave a woman with a whole new level of self-destructive guilt and self-loathing.

Interestingly, Amanda never became pregnant but chose instead to adopt siblings who were already seven and nine years old at the time. While it was not at all the plan she had initially envisioned for herself, Amanda made her choices from a place of inner peace, and joyfully took on her new role as mother. Donna turned in desperation to a fertility specialist that she promised herself would be her last attempt, regardless of whether he could help her or not. Her doctor listened to her tearful account of previous attempts to conceive, and accurately gauged the frustration in her voice. Gently, he helped her realize, "Sometimes, no matter how much you want something, no matter how hard you try, there are some things that are simply outside of your control."

For Donna, the doctor's words were the right message, at the right time. The following year, she gave birth to a little girl. Whether her pregnancy occurred because of the treatments she received from her doctor, because she "unblocked" her own pathway to fertility by taking the pressure off herself, or whether she finally received the benefits of the visualization she had done, no one can say for sure. Perhaps Donna simply became pregnant because it was the right time in her life for her to conceive a child.

Finding Your Feelings

In your quiet space, you may also want to replay events and spend time thinking through how you really feel about them. You can look for the signals your body is sending you about the feelings you are having. You can cry…and you can stop crying.

There is no protocol for how you conduct yourself within your private space. There are no "shoulds" and "shouldn'ts" about what you think, feel, or say aloud. Just as importantly, this is also the place where you do not have to think at all, where you can just "check out," and savor the peace that comes from not talking, not analyzing, and not trying to figure out everything, or anything. But there may be times when you feel blocked, or instances when you wrestle with challenging emotions that are difficult to put into words. At times like these, it is helpful to have guidelines for identifying and processing what you are feeling.

Sometimes you may want your quiet time to be about getting in touch with your feelings, to help you gain perspective, or just to help you find your way to acceptance. Breathing exercises can be helpful in this regard. Chapter 4, "Making Conscious Choices," discussed using your body as a barometer for what is happening emotionally, noticing perhaps the tightness in your chest, or that queasy feeling in your belly.

You can use your quiet time to explore fully the messages your body sends you. Let yourself breathe into your feelings, fully and completely. Keep in mind that, "whatever you resist, persists," so notice your feelings in your body and move toward them with your breath. As emotions rise to the surface, breathe into them and let them wash over you. In this way, you allow yourself to move toward clarity and resolution.

Recall that your body has a language all its own, and you have already learned how an awareness of the three body zones can help you clarify your feelings. These zones represent parts of the body that express primary emotional experiences: fear and anger (the upper back, shoulders, neck); sadness and longing (the throat and chest); and anxiety and nervousness (the stomach). Knowing where in your body emotions seem to manifest can help you identify and give voice to your feelings. Practice sitting in your quiet space, and taking long, slow, deep breaths. Being present to the areas of the body where emotional expression manifests can oftentimes be the key to crystallizing and processing your feelings in a way that enables you to give words to them.

There are times however, when even feedback from your body can feel muddled and confusing. At other times, you may simply want to be more direct in your exploration of what is happening to you emotionally. In his book, *Emotion-Focused Therapy: Coaching Clients to Work Through Their Feelings,* Dr. Leslie Greenberg recommends five steps that prompt you to ask yourself specific questions to get things moving. Try these steps, adapted from Dr. Greenberg's book, any time you are journaling about events that have caused you emotional stress. Take your time, think about your answers, and then record them in your journal.

Step 1.   Is your experience best described by an emotion or feeling word, or by a word that describes a desire to take action in some way?

Step 2.   What is the situation to which you are reacting? Is it an actual event, an internal experience, or another person?

Step 3.   What are the thoughts accompanying this emotion?

(Here, you can use your language of truth in determining what you are imagining or assuming; the story you are telling yourself about a certain situation.)

Step 4. What need, goal, or concern is not being met in this situation?

Step 5. What is your primary emotional experience?

Follow the answers to each of these questions by breathing into your body's experience of your emotion. Use your breathing to let your feelings wash over you, totally and completely.

Your Emotional Messengers

Emotions communicate important messages, and in order to gain clarity, it is helpful for you to stay with the emotional experience you are having until you understand what the feeling is trying to tell you. In fact, Dr. Greenberg believes this is especially true with feelings of sadness and loss. Since these feelings in particular are an inescapable part of the emotional cycle of infertility, pay special attention to ways to process them. The old proverb, "the only way out is through," is certainly true when it comes to dealing with your emotions, and to that end, it is important to give yourself permission to enter into your feelings.

The following exercise provides a meditative experience that can help you when you are struggling with feelings of sadness and loss. Again, this excerpt is an adaptation from Dr. Greenberg's work in *Emotion-Focused Therapy: Coaching Clients to Work Through Their Feelings*.

Slow down, focus on your abdomen, and breathe deeply. Focus on, and let yourself feel your sadness. Identify your loss.

Let yourself feel what this means to you. Tell yourself what it is you miss.

Ask yourself: "What is this emotion communicating to me?" Just feel the feelings and wait. Don't try to analyze or

> *the old proverb, 'the only way out is through,' is certainly true when it comes to dealing with your emotions*

figure it out. Just stay with the physical experience of your feeling. Breathe into your experience, and stay with it until you feel a shift—you are able to relax, or you feel the tears come. Stay with the tears and your sadness until you feel complete for now. Let your tears relax you.

Asking the Right Questions

When you are ready to delve deeper, posing questions to yourself is a wonderful way, not only to process your feelings, but also to help you in decision-making. If you find you are confused and unable to discern your authentic feelings, ask a question of yourself and see what comes to you. But in order to get the best answer, it's important that first you learn to ask the right question.

The importance of asking yourself the right questions comes from the teachings of Dr. Gay Hendricks. At a Hendricks Institute seminar several years ago, Dr. Hendricks spoke of the transformative power of asking "big questions," and how these questions help you draw out of your experiences, the answers that can truly make a difference. The key is in the type of questions you choose to ask.

> *the truth is, why questions are essentially unanswerable, at least in a way that provides any real satisfaction*

Right now, listen to your mental chatter. You will notice that the mind is always asking and answering questions. Even though questions come in all different forms, like who, what, when, or where, one type of question is habitual in human nature—the question *why*.

If you are like most people, you naturally gravitate toward why questions in an attempt to figure out things. But remember, the part of your brain that produces solutions is only about as large as a quarter and even highly intelligent people operate by using only a very small portion of their brain. Don't rely on drawing every answer to every question from within your own head.

The truth is, *why* questions are essentially unanswerable, at least in a way that provides any real satisfaction. Nevertheless, they can keep your mind busy, with possibilities circling endlessly. *Why* questions, along with the stress of trying to figure things out, are exhausting. They represent the very type of thinking that will keep you locked in your issue with no resolution or even forward motion.

Try learning something new with your muscles tight, your breathing tense, and your brain preoccupied with asking *why*. If you're doing everything you can to get pregnant and it's still not happening, *why* questions won't bring you any answers. In fact, *why* questions may be the block preventing you from recognizing new information that really could be helpful.

Melissa, for example, was stuck in her anger about the futility of her efforts to get pregnant. Try as she might, she often felt as if she were on the edge of a downward spiral, berating herself for having waited so long to try to have a baby. At thirty-five years old, Melissa felt as if her most fertile years were behind her, and her self-talk usually played along the tormenting lines of, "Why, why, why did I wait so long?"

The problem was that no matter how often Melissa asked this question, she came no closer to an answer. Sure, she could come up with reasons that she delayed trying to get pregnant, such as a lack of education about her own fertility, or her commitment to her career. But Melissa made the best decisions she could with the information she had at the time. Most importantly, no matter how many *why* questions she asks, she cannot access the information she needs to move forward in her goal to become a mother.

Einstein once said, "Problems cannot be solved at the same level of consciousness that created them." This means if the, "why can't I get preg-nant right now?" question recreates the same feelings of fear and anger that infertility itself creates, then it becomes virtually impossible to access new information and move toward resolution of the question.

What to do?

One of the best ways to access the universe of possibilities is to start paying attention to the questions you ask. The mere act of reconstructing your questions has the power to move you onto the threshold of possibili-ties, and takes you out of the closed room of limitations.

For example, ask yourself the question, "Why can't I get pregnant right now?" Or ask a question that expresses a similar struggle and notice how you feel. Do you observe constriction in your breathing and tightness in your body, perhaps emotions of anger or frustration? Is there a victim-like quality that comes with the question, as in, "Why me?" Can you imagine trying to find answers from this place? This would be the equivalent of walking through life with blinders on, unable to be open to the opportuni-ties around you.

Now watch what happens when you change this *why* question to a *how* or a *what* question. Possibilities like, "What can I do to increase my chances to become pregnant?" may bring to mind the need to get informa-tion on the role of lifestyle or diet, or may prompt you to consider another medical option. Questions such as, "How can I get the emotional support I need right now?" may motivate you to find out more information about the fertility support group flyer you keep seeing at your doctor's office, or to plan to have lunch with a friend who understands your situation.

Notice too, what occurs physically when you change from *why* to *how*. Do you feel more relaxed, open, and expansive? Do you find you stand up a little straighter, almost as if you are more receptive to what is in your environment? Asking the right questions literally opens your perception to the world around you, and to the people, places, and circumstances that can bring you information, clarity, and the possibility of resolution.

Once you begin to pay attention and look at what's around you through the lens of your new questions, you will be amazed at the ways in which new information will find you. You might be standing in a checkout line and overhear a conversation that fills in a gap you've been searching to fill. Or perhaps you'll be flipping channels on the TV, and just happen to land on a talk show that is discussing the very issue about which you were wondering. Or a friend will rave about a new book that speaks to the subject that's been on your mind. Life can be very creative when it comes to answering your questions if you just know the right questions to ask. When you are open to it, answers to your personal questions flow not only from inside your head out into the world, but also from the collective wisdom of the universe, straight into your heart.

Quite simply, *why* is always a question about where you have been, in other words, about the past. But *how* and *what* are questions about where you are going. Whether or not you have a medical diagnosis, you may never know the *why* of your present struggle. Like Melissa, you too, may not be able to undo a choice you made in the past. But asking the right questions can allow you to focus on what you need in your life to best take you where you want to go, given where you are now.

Going through this process and transforming your questions is a great way to get unstuck and become more empowered. If you notice you are having difficulty transforming your *whys* into more effective questions, it is a good indication that you are stuck in your old way of thinking. Be aware that clearing away resistance may take a little work, so have patience with yourself. Use your journal to explore the blocks holding your back and the negative self-talk that may be blocking you. Once you are able to gain clarity in this way, it becomes much easier to define a new direction and to be able consciously to choose beliefs and thoughts that will help you move forward.

This leads to another way your journal can be helpful in accessing the wisdom inside you. Next time you need an answer, just write your question and then spend a moment taking a couple of slow, deep breaths and trying to clear your mind. Begin writing whatever comes into your head. Write without thinking and let the words come tumbling out. Often, it is amazing to discover the wisdom that lies dormant and is waiting for an opportunity to be expressed.

Quite simply, asking the right question is the challenging part. Once you are clear on the question, the answers, whether they come quickly and easily or slowly over time, will often take care of themselves. In the words of Rainer Maria Rilke, in his book, *Letters to a Young Poet,* "Don't search for answers…Live the questions now. Perhaps then, you will gradually, without even noticing it, live your way into the answer."

Re-entering the Larger Room

Taking quiet space is powerful. It allows you to have an outlet for your feelings so that you are able to gain clarity and discover what needs to happen next. As you prepare to make your transition from the quiet space of your small room, into the larger room of the rest of your world, ask yourself, "What do I need right now, to heal, and to move forward?" Just ask the question, and then wait and see what comes.

After giving yourself time to sit with your feelings, you may discover that you need to make a place within yourself to accept loving attention, a gentle touch or a warm hug from someone who is willing to be there for you—your husband or a close friend. You may realize that you need to pay more attention to the way you speak to yourself, using language that provides encourage-

 it's not that the goal is to never get off track, but to get off less often, less intensively, and for shorter periods of time

ment and affirmation. Sometimes you may feel you need to mark the end of your quiet time with a simple ritual that provides a sense of acknowledgement or completion, and that allows you to let go, even if just a little, and make space for something new. Whatever this special place opens for you and however this time guides you, be grateful for the inner wisdom that is waiting when you simply make the choice to step into your own quiet space.

FROM MARINA'S CASE FILES ON

Leslie C.

religion means different things to everyone. But there are some, like Leslie, who believe if they, "do everything right" they will be protected from disappointment and heartache. Unfortunately, life doesn't come with guarantees.

Leslie, age twenty-nine, was the classic "good girl." Raised a Christian, she took her faith to heart, and "did everything right." She was a virgin when she got married, and has lived what she described as an "upright, Christian life." Leslie described her husband as very loving, but unfortunately, she related that he had a hard time providing her with the emotional support she needed, trying to rationalize and fix, rather than just listen. Even talking to her pastor proved fruitless, and Leslie continued to feel alone and misunderstood. After some soul searching, Leslie was able to acknowledge that she was "angry and feeling betrayed by God." It was almost as if she was saying, "We made a deal, God, and you're not keeping your end of the bargain." Of course, this only caused Leslie to feel even more guilty and isolated, trapping her in a vicious cycle.

Leslie's fertility treatment experience, as she moved through several trials of unsuccessful IUI's, (intra-uterine inseminations) essentially became a spiritual crisis. Even her job, acting as a case manager for child abuse and neglect cases, served as a reminder of her belief that God doesn't play fair. As a result, much of her work with me centered around maturing spiritually. Leslie needed to "grow up" her relationship with God, from that of a child believing that a parental God will reward her for good behavior, to a mature adult accepting that, when "bad things happen," even to good people, spirituality can be a source of strength and solace.

Following some precepts of the 12-Step Program proved very helpful for Leslie. She realized that despite her former claims of trusting in a loving God, she came to see that her "good behavior" was really a way for her to try to manipulate God to do her will. She also acknowledged that her addictions to perfectionism and control are what truly made her life unmanageable, and that she needed to surrender her will, and this process, over to that of a loving God. Adopting a basic precept of the 12-Step Programs, she learned to take it "one day at a time."

Spending quiet time and journaling was particularly helpful in this process. Journaling in particular provided Leslie with the opportunity to "write letters to God," and honor her feelings of anger, loss, even longing. Over time, she noticed a shift, and spiritually she began to heal and grow. Through her journaling, she was also able to acknowledge her need for the support of other women, and this led to her involvement in a local infertility support group, where she built deep, meaningful relationships with other women. Her ongoing commitment to the strength of this support was pivotal in contributing to the local growth of this community.

Before undergoing what was to be her final IUI, Leslie discovered she was pregnant. Her joy was matched by the realization that this journey had also allowed her the opportunity to truly grow her spiritual relationship with God. She learned the importance of letting go of her own agenda, and living more from a place of spontaneity and trust.

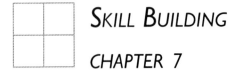

SKILL BUILDING

CHAPTER 7

1. In the case file of Leslie C., you read about her success in using her journal effectively, including writing letters to God. As you explore journaling, select a relationship that you find occupies your thoughts frequently. Try letter writing as a way to increase your own understanding of your feelings, regardless of whether your letter is to God, or as the chapter suggested, to your "spouse or partner, the child you have not conceived, your doctor, your mother, or even your spirit guide." Your letter might also be to yourself as a child or your future self. Write and just be open to what your letter tells you about your feelings.

2. *Asking the right questions...*

    Listen in on your self-talk, and write down two *why* questions you have asked yourself more than three times. Now redesign these questions so that they shift into *how* or *what* questions.

    Sit with one of your new questions. Notice how you feel physically. Breathe into this. Observe if there is any new information that you are able to access. If there is, decide on one step you can take to step into this answer. If you can't yet take a step, that's okay. Simply make a choice to pay attention to whatever comes into your experience.

3. *Letting it go...*

    If you've been carrying around sadness and loss, now's a good time to honor it and let go. Set aside one of your quiet time sessions for specifically this purpose, and write about your pain and sorrow. Stay awake to your breathing throughout, and let your feelings be what they are. Then, when you feel complete for now, light a candle and burn what you have written. As you watch the smoke disappear, make a conscious intention to let go of all you have been carrying.

Your Sixth Power Tool: Give Yourself Permission to Grieve

Feelings are neither good, nor bad. They just are.
You've been reading this statement since Chapter 3, but as a concept, it is a difficult one to grasp. As information you take ownership of and apply to your own life, it can be an extremely challenging idea.

Feelings or emotions are byproducts of living. Your experiences create the texture, color, and variety in the tapestry of your life. Your emotions are, in a sense, you communicating with yourself about your experiences. But you are not your emotions. Your emotions are separate from the part of you that has the power to stand separate from those feelings and notice what is being evoked for you, to run your hand over the complex and exquisite texture of your life's tapestry, scrutinizing it to take in all the colors, variations, and nuances. Some of the fabric of your life will feel rough to the touch, while other patches will be silky smooth. Some of the colors will be vibrant and splendid, others muted and peaceful, some drab, and others will simply clash or be downright ugly.

your sixth power tool is: give yourself permission to grieve

This is your life and it is beautiful in its own distinctive way. Your challenge comes in learning to see it as lovely and to love it because it belongs to you and you alone. Ironically, the parts of the fabric that are fine and smooth are often the most fragile, while the parts that are rough and coarse are usually the strongest. You could attempt to weave a monochromatic bolt of endlessly matching fabric, but who really wants to look back at the end of her days and say, "I kept my emotions as limited as possible by deliberately participating in life as little as I could"?

You fall into a trap if you assume that life would be best if you are happy 365 days each year and the fabric of your life is seamless. Think about it. If you were sublimely happy every day, day after day, would happiness still *feel* like happiness? The answer is no, because you would not have a basis for comparison. Like eating ice cream for breakfast, lunch and dinner, seven days a week for the rest of your existence, life on an ice cream-only diet would not only bore you, it could quickly turn into little more than sugar overload interrupted by occasional episodes of painful brain freeze.

Continual happiness, like endless-ice cream, is not a realistic, sustainable, or even necessarily desirable objective. When it comes to conceiving a child, there is only one way to guarantee that you can avoid the pain of infertility and that is to never attempt to have a child and never, ever let yourself think about motherhood and family life. If you do not pursue motherhood, then you won't have to face disappointment if it never happens to you.

But that ship has already sailed. The good news is that you would not have wanted to be onboard anyway. Living an emotionally pain-free life would not only include never trying to conceive in order to avoid risking failure, it would include other avoidances, such as never loving someone because the object of your affection might die, leave you, or stop returning your love. In fact, the only foolproof way to limit your experience of unpleasant emotions is to stop interacting with other people entirely, and even then, you risk feelings like loneliness and a sense of isolation.

The moment you began thinking about conceiving a child, you opened yourself up to experiencing great happiness. You also opened life up to new avenues that lead to varying degrees of painful, disappointing, and frustrating emotions. You could fail to conceive a child at all. You could be successful in having a child only to face challenging situations down the road. The possibilities for new and unfamiliar emotions become wide open the moment you introduce a new objective or new direction into your goals.

Of course, fear of failure and a desire to avoid painful emotions should never stop you from rolling the dice and moving forward in your life toward your realistic and achievable desires. Yet neither should you set yourself up for guaranteed failure, by expecting the words "happily ever after," to be embroidered across every event you experience. To live fully means to accept that life comes with a full range of emotions. If you try to cut yourself off from one emotion or another, your whole experience of life can become stagnant and compromised.

Grief, for example, encapsulates a wide range of emotional experiences, including the denial, anger, and sadness that are inherent in the diagnosis of infertility. If you are undergoing fertility treatments, you will find that both the chemical and the psychological effects of the treatments leave your emotions tuned to an unusually high-pitch. This is challenging, but you can remind yourself that the emotions you feel also come from what you are communicating to yourself about your infertility experience, and in this way, you do have some choices.

Having choices is particularly important because the grief of infertility is ongoing, and alternates from the highs of anticipating that this time things work, to the crushing loss from a failed procedure, or another disappointing menstrual cycle. This pattern is exhausting and it is *critical* that you use all the tools you have thus far packed in your toolbox to help turn down the volume on the high-pitched emotions you are feeling. As you read this chapter you will see how you need to apply the tools of caring for your body, making conscious choices, setting healthy boundaries, telling the truth, and taking quiet space in order to give yourself permission to grieve. But the first important part of the grieving experience comes with giving yourself adequate time.

Rethink the Way You Look at Time

Time management advice is available everywhere. Suggestions for managing time fill the pages of books and magazines. You can go online and find e-books, seminars, articles, and blogs dedicated to the topic of teaching you better methods for managing your time. But time does not change; it never speeds up and it never slows down. By its very nature, time defies management. To complicate this idea further, you also have to face the fact that you cannot ultimately control life, either. Life happens, and in the process, things just occur. You can enhance your chances of being handed good things and diminish your chances of being handed bad things by making good choices, but you still cannot control the intrinsically uncontrollable aspects of life. You can do everything possible to ensure fertility; nonetheless, it may still elude you. The only aspect of your world over which you have any genuine control, is in *how you choose to respond to the events life dishes out.*

Throw out arbitrary timelines that called for you to have a baby by the time you were thirty, thirty-five, or forty. Whatever script you took your ideas from is just that—a script you wrote for yourself or you let others write for you. You do not have to have a child at any predetermined time, or even to have a child at all, in order to experience a rich and meaningful life. Think about how much less emotionally painful fertility treatment would be if you were truly convinced that, despite how much you want to have a child, *your life would still be wonderful whether or not it ever happens?* Or that *if you truly want a family, it will happen, even though it may look and feel different from what you imagine?*

Rather than barreling ahead to meet self-imposed timelines, take a break whenever your body signals that you need one. Take time off between cycles to grieve, regroup, and recoup. Do not try to be Wonder Woman. Your doctor, your spouse, or your best friend do not know and understand what you are personally experiencing. If you feel overwhelmed, it is because you *are* overwhelmed. That feedback from your emotions needs to stand alone, and to be enough motivation for you to do what is right for you.

Knowing When Enough Is Enough

The quest to conceive a child takes women from the intimacy of their bedrooms to the sterile environment of medical laboratories. Once you get there, it can be, in a sense, very difficult to figure out when to leave and where to go if you do leave. If only your doctor would say, "it is time to stop treatments." But of course, doctors rarely take the responsibility of making that decision for patients. Even when they do state that everything medically possible has been done at this time and the couple should consider other ways of building a family, a patient may be very unreceptive to hearing and internalizing the doctor's words. In a process that builds one hope on top of another hope, it can be extremely difficult for many women to hear, "there is no more hope."

If you haven't already done so, now is a good time to consider using *outcome based thinking* to help you with your decision-making. Kevin Hogan is the author of *The Psychology of Persuasion*, a book that has been published in more than eight languages. In *The Psychology of Persuasion*, Hogan explains outcome based thinking as a simple strategy that allows you to know how far you are willing to go toward a certain objective. For example, before you enter into negotiations with a new car dealer, outcome based thinking calls for you to decide that you will buy the Camry you want only if the dealer agrees to a price that is less than $21,000 and he has a vehicle in stock that is blue with an automatic transmission. Outcome based thinking enables you to know before you enter the car purchasing process, precisely what you want the outcome of your efforts to be. You know at what point you will make the decision to buy or to walk away. The process of selecting and negotiating to purchase a car becomes clearly easier because you have given yourself a measure of control, despite the fact that you have no control at all over what the car dealer does or says.

Having a child feels like a very different type of life decision than whether or not to buy a new car, and in some regards, it is. However, in many ways, the bottom line of most situations in life comes down to acknowledging only the options you actually can control. Even when you are facing emotion-driven life issues, you will benefit tremendously from applying basic principles of decision-making.

When you are dealing with the challenges of infertility, your first thought may be, "Duh, I will stop trying to conceive *when* I get pregnant." *But what will you do if the dealer does not have that blue Camry priced less than $21,000 on his lot?*

At some point, you can't just continue to walk around the car lot, hoping a blue Camry will turn up. You have to go home and get on with your life. You may later decide to keep driving your old Corolla. You may decide you will go with a green Camry or a blue Mustang, but whatever you decide, you can't devote the rest of your life to the hope that someday a blue Camry will appear on the car lot at the price you are willing to pay. Wanting something with all your heart may seem as if it should be enough to make that something happen, but the reality is—*it's not!*

> *wanting something with all your heart may seem as if it should be enough to make that something happen, but the reality is,* it's not

Conceiving a child is certainly the outcome you hope to achieve as you deal with your fertility challenges, but you need to know, for your own sake, that if it doesn't happen, there is a time and a place when this effort will stop being the center of your life. Knowing when you will stop is one of the few areas of control you have in the whole fertility-infertility experience. Don't give it up!

Step up to the control that is possible for you and at the same time let go of your attempts to control the aspects that are never going to be within your power to direct. Try to decide as early as possible in your fertility challenge just how far you are willing to go. Create a set point that clearly communicates, "I will not go beyond this specific marker to pursue conception of a baby." Your set point may be a work in progress that takes months or years to establish. You may base it on a predetermined number of treatments. Using a dollar figure can be a very realistic way to determine when to say, "I have had enough."

Establishing your set point puts control back in your hands. A predetermined set point tells you and your spouse or partner when you will be turning the page and taking your life in a new direction. Be prepared that the two of you may not see eye-to-eye on where and when to set the stopping point. What are the odds you will share the same perception of when your set point should be? But if you and your spouse do not work through this issue together, in a way that is mutually respectful of each other, then deciding when you will stop your efforts will cause new resentments to develop and become a whole new point of conflict within your marriage.

As you make your decision, think of your marriage as involving three considerations: what is right for you; what your husband or partner feels is right for him; and what is right for the marriage. When "the marriage" takes on an identity of its own, marital compromise often becomes much easier.

Suppose your husband says, "We cannot borrow more than fifty thousand dollars against our home to pay for fertility treatments." Even though you agree with him from a financial perspective, you may find it difficult to put a dollar value on your desire to have a child. You may think it is inappropriate to correlate a baby with a budget, believing that having a child is worth any financial sacrifice. But step back from your situation and ask yourself what would happen to the stability of the marriage (the third entity that must be considered) if instead of fifty thousand dollars of debt, the marriage was faced with a debt of one hundred thousand, incurred in the pursuit of conceiving a child? How would this added burden of debt affect—not you—not your husband—but "the marriage"? Would the marriage still be strong enough to sustain the two of you as good parents and good spouses if one or both of you were forced to take a second job? Would your ability to parent be diminished if you had to sell your house and return to living in an apartment, a house trailer, or with your parents or in-laws? And what happens if you create thousands of dollars in debt and there is still no baby? Sometimes it is actually a good thing that the money for fertility treatments is limited, because it can stand as a clear road marker for when it is time for a couple to take a different path.

Perhaps for you and your spouse, money is no object. Even if you have unlimited funds to devote to the pursuit of a pregnancy, you must still consider the strain the process places on each of you. The days, months, or years you are devoting to achieving a pregnancy, and the way this pursuit leaves your life in a constant state of limbo, are a price you pay. Consider what your pursuit of pregnancy is costing you in funds, time, energy, and emotional debt.

Couples who learn to put the needs of the marriage before their individual objectives build strong marriages. The skills they develop in dealing with the stresses created by their fertility challenge carry them through and over other types of pitfalls that come their way. Honoring the needs of "the marriage" demands unselfish decision-making on the part of both the husband and the wife.

An important detail to consider about establishing a set point for when to stop fertility treatments is that your decision must *always* include the option for you to take "vacations" from the treatment process. If at any time, your fertility treatments become too stressful for your mind or body to handle, you must allow yourself the opportunity to take a timeout or stop them entirely, even if you have not yet reached your set point. Throughout both the treatment and the process of determining your set point, it is important to keep the doors of communication open, and keep checking in with yourself and with your spouse.

Why Quitting is So Hard

Giving birth to a child is not just about social and personal conditioning and expectations. Bearing children is coded within your DNA. Spring romance and mating season are all part of an elaborate structure that ensures survival of the species. No matter how sophisticated a culture becomes, no one is insulated from the primal instinct to bear young.

There are many aspects to the complex desire to have a child of your own. To some degree, people want children because they seek to rewrite their own lives. They want to give a child everything they had that was good and everything they did not have but longed to experience or own. You may justifiably feel that you and your spouse or partner would make incredible parents, but your longing to have that child has nothing to do with the child herself, (who does not exist yet) and everything to do with how you feel about being a parent to that still as yet, *imaginary* child.

If you think it through objectively, which is understandably very hard to do, you will discover that your desire to have a child is entirely about you. The fact that having a child is a self-centered objective does not make it selfish, wrong, or bad. But it is helpful if you can see your desire from an honest perspective.

The possibility of life without a child forces you into other levels of thinking. You begin to question if your marriage is good enough to be sufficiently fulfilling without children. You may wonder if your personality is enough to enjoy, enrich, and entertain your spouse and *yourself* without the addition of a child. You will have other questions as well, like, whether you will still have friendships if all your friends have children and you don't. Or whether, as you and your husband grow older, will you be lonely without children?

If you can begin to explore some of your questions, you will also find a measure of perspective about your experience with infertility. This perspective will allow you to find answers about what you really want. For example, do you want pregnancy or do you want parenthood? Gaining perspective allows you to acknowledge the repercussions of whatever choice you make. It increases your chances of finding peace and contentment with yourself, and helps give you the strength to make the best decisions, no matter what life hands you.

You Haven't Failed

Human beings are competitive by instinct. When there are no other players in the field, people still compete against themselves. And almost everyone is willing to compete against Mother Nature.

As you go through your efforts to conceive a child, periodically pause and check with yourself to make sure that your diligent pursuit of your goal is still about motherhood, and hasn't just become about "winning". Wanting to beat the odds, slay the leviathan, or win the prize of a baby are all natural ways to feel while you are in the process of trying to conceive. You've put a great deal of time, money, and effort into achieving your goal and it makes sense that you want results. You want to move outside the ranks of childless couples and into what you perceive to be the winner's circle. You may feel that good people seeking well-intentioned results inevitably are rewarded or that when you pay a price, you *earn* certain results.

Stopping or giving up on your quest is hard, especially when there is always the thought that the next procedure might be "the one". Hope is addictive. Today's culture admonishes you if you are a quitter. Media messages bombard you, telling you to envision your putts or basketballs dropping into the cylinder and they will; to see yourself as thin, and the pounds will start to come off; or to set career goals and envision yourself achieving them. If you want to stop smoking, drinking, or overspending, you can find plenty of support and advice. But where do you turn for a role

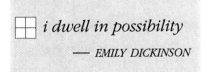

i dwell in possibility

— *EMILY DICKINSON*

model when you set out to quit a worthwhile effort? There are virtually no media messages that guide you to be a quitter in a pursuit that is positive or considered to be a good thing. Today's world praises victory through persistence and determination. In a culture that communicates that believing hard enough will give you the power to achieve any goal, it is easy to begin to identify with the triumphant 1980 US Olympic hockey team or any other successful champion who started out as the underdog and defied the odds.

The feeling that you are giving up or quitting is very scary. Loss or failure in one area of your life feels as if it has the power to infiltrate other areas. It doesn't! Stopping your fertility treatments does not have to mean that your time and efforts were wasted. As much as you may feel that you have undergone your experience in a vacuum, you have not. Your life has touched the lives of many other people and right now, you may not even realize that you have helped, healed, or influenced someone else in a meaningful way. Even more importantly, your experience with infertility changes both you and your partner forever. Each of you can choose to view and process this experience in a positive way, and in so doing, reap the rewards this life passage offers.

Grief is Good

Staying involved in fertility treatment perpetuates a grief cycle that is unique in nature—up one day, and down the next. But once you make the decision to end treatment, it becomes necessary to bury your "never-born child" and move on. This is challenging because in dealing with the loss of the never-born child, you can struggle to identify when hope ends and grieving begins.

Women who experience the death of a child, begin to grieve the moment the child ceases to breathe. This loss is unimaginable, it is wrenching beyond words, but there is finality to it, an identifiable end.

Yet the loss of your longed-for child can be just as real, just as poignant, because a child is born in your heart long before it ever takes form. Marina works with many women who have been so invested in their vision of a child that they actually carry within them a mental image of who *he* will look like, or what *she* will become. But this very thing that sustained hope during infertility treatment is the loss that must be acknowledged and grieved in order to heal. As difficult as this is, grieving the loss of this never-born child is essential. Grief is a gateway, a threshold, over which you must step in order to gain clarity and eventually acceptance. Infertility will always be a part of your history, but whether or not you eventually find resolution and make peace as you move forward has a lot to do with how you handle your grief now.

For centuries, people in most cultures marked their period of grief in very public ways. The well-known Roman toga was not just the popular form of dress. Togas symbolized Roman citizenship and the wearing of one was an honor. While the image of the Roman man in his white toga is well known, togas in other colors signified specific types of events. Following the death of a family member or close friend, or during a period of danger or distress, Roman citizens wore the *toga pulla*, a dark woolen garment that communicated to others this was a person in mourning.

Over the years, most cultures have set standards of specific dress and behavior during times of mourning. Sometimes mourning dress was white, but most typically it was black or dark in color. Other customs have included wearing a locket that contains a photograph of the deceased or lock of his or her hair, wearing veils to mask your face, flying a flag at half-staff, and other practices that visually communicate grief both to the person who is mourning and to the rest of the world. Such efforts are important because they demonstrate that a person is acknowledging her grief and living through a time in her life that is markedly different from the periods that precede and follow it. A woman in mourning communicates to others that she should be treated with an extra measure of consideration. Just as significantly, she communicates to herself in a very concrete way that she is experiencing the emotion of grief and she is not running from it. Instead of avoiding her grief, she is putting it on like a garment; she is literally stepping into the emotion.

In recent years, many people have taken a John Wayne approach to grieving. Being stoic has become admirable. Grieving individuals often strive to act in such a way that people remark as to how well they are handling their tragedy or to give the appearance that they are unaffected by the sad event. Shock, denial, even repression of feelings has been mistaken for strength. In the meantime, all that unresolved loss festers within, blocking the way to clarity, to hope, to creating a new life. Truly, there is no gain by failing to cry, failing to mourn, and pretending to be okay with something about which you do not feel okay at all.

Historically, periods of grieving have extended for months and even years. In nineteenth century England, women mourned for up to four years following the death of a child or spouse. Jewish tradition recognizes the one year anniversary of a death as a *yahrzeith* (year time) and observes memorials or special services to acknowledge the period of mourning and grief. Time is important in the grieving process.

Taking deliberate action to symbolize and process your grief is also a very good thing. You are justifiably sad about going through the experience of infertility. If you do not conceive a child, you are further saddened by the loss of the child you will never bear. While you are not likely to conduct a funeral to memorialize your loss, you may find

grief is a gateway, a threshold, over which you must step in order to gain clarity, and eventually, acceptance

great comfort in doing something that helps you acknowledge your loss and brings closure to this period of your life. Perhaps you and your spouse will plant a tree. Maybe you will write your thoughts on paper and then together cast them into the ocean, or burn them in a campfire, sending your thoughts out into the greater universe, while at the same time changing the way you view them in your present life.

The grieving process is the *only* way out of the oppressive emotions you feel after a loss. When someone you love dies, you never stop missing that person and you never stop feeling his or her loss. But as you have observed in others or in yourself, as time passes and you become more acclimated to your loss, you begin to live with it more comfortably.

Do not shut down grief. Move into it and embrace it. Back away from your usual routine and give yourself a less demanding schedule and more private time to be alone and allow yourself to feel your emotions. Because you are not experiencing a loss that others see in the way they see a death of a loved one, no one will be sending you cards of consolation or flowers to show their sympathy. Why not buy your own fresh flowers? Place them on your desk or bedside table. Find your own ways to acknowledge and even memorialize your experience, whether you do it privately or you share it in some ways with others. Take time in your quiet space every day to sit with your memories, with your feelings of loss. Journal about what comes up for you. Honor this time of mourning in your life, and allow yourself to accept the help of those who love and care about you.

The Power of Ritual

nothing can bring you peace but yourself"
— RALPH WALDO EMERSON

Throughout history, religious traditions have utilized the power of ritual to honor an event or mark a passage. But rites of this nature do not have to be limited to formal settings. You can also create your own ritual to give expression to your grief.

In her book, *Grief Unseen: Healing Pregnancy Loss Through the Arts,* author Laura Seftel notes, "rituals provide a focal point of awareness that we are moving through an obstacle, transitioning to a new sense of self, or letting go of something lost…Rituals allow us…to create connections with ourselves, each other, and our experience of the sacred."

The simple act of lighting a candle or planting a tree can be rich with significance. A ceremony can be pivotal as you journey to acceptance. Your ceremony can be performed on your own or with others, and may include personal mementos, the elements of nature, or symbols that reflect your spiritual beliefs.

Support from Others

When you are grieving or mourning a loss, there is comfort in the human touch. Schedule time to let other people nurture you and take care of your needs. Get a manicure or a massage. Let your hairdresser shampoo your hair. Even though you may not immediately recognize the benefits, human touch is extremely healing. If you typically benefit from acupuncture or even just enjoy something as simple as the way your mouth feels after the dental hygienist cleans your teeth, then now is the time to schedule such treatments and let others help take care of you physically.

Fertility support groups are also a valuable way to help you to deal with your feelings, whether you are still in treatment, or are exploring whether it's time to shift gears. Support groups allow you to know that you are not alone, and they give you a place to share your feelings, fears, and experiences with people who genuinely understand. Fertility support groups can be an enormous source of comfort and guidance. These groups, which are based within your community or are available through your local medical community or organizations like RESOLVE, offer the most direct route to a support network, as well as a path to new friendships. There is nothing like sharing your story to let you know that you are not alone.

Your grief about your infertility experience or about a child you will not have, may last much longer than you (or people around you) think it should. There are no "shoulds" about what is right when it comes to grieving. You and your spouse or partner will not experience the grief of infertility in the same way, nor will you work through it on the same schedule.

Because your grief is less tangible to others than it would be if you, for example, were experiencing the death of your three-year-old child, other people may not be as responsive and as sensitive to your feelings. Caught up in their own lives friends, family members, or co-workers may not acknowledge that you have any reason to grieve at all. Or they may want to comfort you, but be embarrassed or confused about what is the right thing to do or say.

Sometimes their efforts to console you will frustrate you, even though you may not realize exactly why. People who tell you, "I'm sorry," or "Please tell me if I can help," are giving you support in a way that usually feels comforting. People who say to you, "This is God's will," or "Everything happens for a reason," are well intentioned, but you may find that their comments irritate you or leave you feeling even more upset. Try to learn to take both the well chosen and the ill-chosen words only for what they are meant to be: *attempts to offer you comfort.*

Also keep in mind what you learned in Chapter 4, and don't be afraid to back away from people who, unintentionally say the wrong thing and bring all your painful feelings back to the surface. While it is not healthy to become a hermit during your time of grieving, do not hesitate to set boundaries with people or situations that increase your level of stress.

Time to reflect on your emotions and sort through your feelings privately does not mean cutting yourself off from the world. The internet offers many websites with advice and suggestions for dealing with fertility, as well as the opportunity to interact with other women who are going through fertility challenges themselves. One of the benefits of talking online with other women is that anonymity is very freeing. You may find it far easier to be candid with strangers than you do with your well-meaning friends and family. When you talk about your feelings in chat rooms and online support groups, you can say things and ask questions with the liberating sense that no one can judge you because, across the vast expanse of cyberspace, no one knows who you are. The website www.IAmMore.net is an excellent place to learn, vent, and just reflect on your experience with infertility.

When It's More Than Sadness

If you find you are having symptoms of depression that seem unrelated to the ups and downs of treatment, such as constant sadness, sleeping too much or insomnia, eating too much or too little, feelings of worthlessness, lack of motivation, or withdrawal from social activities, professional counseling may be in order. These symptoms are not just a sign of grieving; they represent genuine depression. Counseling will help you gain insight into your feelings and learn how to communicate more effectively, so you can emerge healthier and stronger. Be sure that the licensed professional you choose for counseling is not only someone with whom you feel comfortable, but also someone who has experience with the grief aspects of infertility and reproductive issues.

Coming Out the Other Side

Outcome-based thinking not only can help you know when to bring closure to your efforts, outcome based thinking can also help you understand when to move out of the grieving period. Because some cultures expected the bereaved to grieve for a year or two, or even four years, the person in mourning had a structure and in a way, a type of control. Obviously, when it comes to how long to grieve, one size does not fit all. At some point, however, you need to set some personal mile markers for when you will begin to move away from your period of mourning. Even with this goal in mind, do not be surprised if you discover that your grief manifests as good days and bad days. Just when you think you are doing better, you will inexplicably find yourself standing in line at Starbucks sobbing or sitting in the boss's Monday morning meeting with tears threatening to spill down your face. Such experiences are normal and happen to everyone who is dealing with a loss. They do not represent a "relapse" or a setback in the grieving process; irregularity is innate in grief.

Part of your grieving process includes recognizing that even though you may not feel better now, there will come a time in the future when your pain is less. In the same way you give yourself a marker to indicate when you are going to stop proactively pursuing a pregnancy, give yourself markers to serve as targets and help remind you that your period of intense grieving will not consume your life forever.

people often gain the most from the very experiences that seem to also take the most away from them

Pick a date in the future and schedule a second honeymoon or a romantic weekend getaway so you and your partner can experience the renewed joy of lovemaking with no other agenda than to be loving, sexual, and intimate. If you have decided to end fertility treatment, and not pursue a pregnancy, you may want to go back on birth control as a way to finalize your decision.

Getting out in nature is enormously restorative, and something as simple as planning a quiet day at the beach or by a lake, can be a way to let some of the emptiness in your heart be filled with the sound of the waves, the babbling of a small stream or the fragrance of wildflowers in bloom. Look for opportunities to expand your own nurturing and creative tendencies. Collect seed catalogues and design a garden you will plant in the spring. Make a plan to work with your grandmother or perhaps the older lady who lives alone next door and learn a skill she knows such as quilting. Let yourself enjoy the process of selecting your fabrics and planning your project. Schedule events you can look forward to and anticipate as positive and pleasurable, and then work toward them. The times in your life when there does not seem to be any light at the end of the tunnel are the times when you are most called upon to send up a flare and move forward by its glow.

In the early stages of your grieving period, you may not feel receptive to change, but as time goes by, making even small changes will be very healing. Take a class you have always wanted to take; cut your hair or dye it a different color. Do things that change your old patterns and open your life to new ideas and experiences. However, do not make drastic changes during your grieving period. Twelve step programs recommend a one-year period for deferring any important decisions, and the wisdom of this time-line can apply here. Your hair will grow back if you, on an impulse, decide to go from shoulder length curls to a super-short bob. But other decisions like quitting a job, leaving your spouse, or even moving across country are not the types of life decisions you want to make during your mourning period when your judgment is naturally distorted by the trauma you have experienced.

In time, the new job, new residence and sometimes even the new marital status, may be just what you need, but put those decisions on the back burner for now. Even if you later make a major change and it proves itself with time to be the right move for you, all life changes—even the good ones—bring stress. The one thing you do not want to do at this point is give yourself added sources of stress.

As you find yourself working through your grief and coming to terms with your feelings about infertility, you will begin seeing your life as more than a microcosmic event building only toward the goal of conception. Grieving the vision of the family you had hoped for makes space for new choices, and eventually, a new vision. Without this process, life becomes a series of default decisions…a limbo of broken dreams and hoped for outcomes never to be. But grief eventually opens the door to acceptance, and acceptance allows you to reclaim and recreate your life.

Have you ever heard cancer survivors speak of the "gifts" that came to them through their experience with the disease? How can a potentially fatal disease in which both the illness and much of the treatment for the illness tortures the body, mind, and spirit, leave anyone to view it as a gift or blessing? Cancer survivors are often able to see beating cancer as the impetus that propelled them into being stronger, more focused, and more empowered individuals. They realize that for the rest of their lives, flowers will smell sweeter, skies will look infinitely bluer, the sounds of laughter will ring out with greater resonance, and every experience, whether good or bad, will be more appreciated, simply because they have been given a second chance in life to experience it. Ironically, people often gain the most from the very experiences that seem to take the most away from them.

Your world is not that microcosm, defined by the presence or absence of a pregnancy. Instead, your experience with infertility is but one event that exists, but does not define the whole of who you are or any of the things you have been given the opportunity to accomplish with your life. But in order to see the gifts and the personal breakthrough that your experience with infertility can bring into your life, you must first cross the grief-threshold. You must turn your vision from the microcosmic to the macrocosmic. You must begin to look at the big picture.

FROM MARINA'S CASE FILES ON

Yolanda M.

Sometimes it's hard to stop something we're really good at, even if that something may be killing us.

Yolanda was born to be a caregiver. The oldest daughter in a large Cuban family, Yolanda carried with her a strong matriarchal legacy defining the role of women. Deeply influenced by her grandmother and her great-aunt, who before passing, had lived with the family since Yolanda was a child, she learned the ways of women in her family. In Yolanda's family, this meant to be the strong one, the one who put everyone else's needs before her own. Yolanda learned too, that despite whatever else you may accomplish, having children was the most important role in a woman's life.

To Yolanda, life began when you got married and had a family. But marriage was a little late in coming into Yolanda's life. So while she was waiting, she became a preschool teacher, relishing the mothering opportunity this role provided. And Yolanda practiced her mothering outside the classroom as well. She was the one *everybody* came to with his or her problems. Colleagues, friends, family members, even parents of her pre-school children, all came to Yolanda. The thing was, Yolanda loved being there for others, loved that relaxed look that crept into people's faces when they realized she was really listening, and loved the attention and validation she got. *So what if she had to forget about her own needs and feelings? So what if she needed to pretend that things were always all right with her?* This was a small price to pay for how important she was to so many people.

When Yolanda married, she assumed her caregiving role would just spill over into the children she would have. But pregnancy in her late thirties did not come quickly, and after a year of trying, Yolanda became distraught. One day, while at work, Yolanda doubled over in pain. Examination by her physician revealed a condition of which she was previously unaware, widespread endometriosis.

Rather than pursue medical treatment, Yolanda continued as before. Over the years, Yolanda had carefully cultivated the defense of denial…denial of her own emotional needs, feelings, and desires. Physical denial was just a short jump from there, and Yolanda refused to acknowledge there might be something wrong with her that would prevent her from a successful pregnancy. As the pain worsened, she used whatever means necessary to help her withstand the pain. Instead of dealing with the issue, she traveled from doctor to doctor, looking for a positive prognosis for a worsening condition. By this time, her endometriosis was spreading to her other internal organs. She was told that the situation was serious and hysterectomy was her only option.

When Yolanda finally turned to counseling, her denial was no longer working. Quite simply, she was devastated, and she needed to come to terms with her grief. For Yolanda, not only was this about her inability to have a child, she was also losing who she thought she was. As she readied herself to undergo a surgery, she was overwhelmed to realize that she would need caregiving and support from others. Never in her life had she been in this position.

Yolanda learned to move in small steps to reclaim parts that had been lost to her. She stopped apologizing for her softness and sentimentality. She sat with her husband and shared the depth of her grief and pain. To her surprise, he didn't flinch, but instead was relieved that she was beginning to acknowledge her pain. She shared with some family members too, not only the enormity of what she felt now, but also how she had never wanted to be a bother, believing this to be the way to their love. Yolanda shared these things not so much because she wanted their validation now, but because she came to realize that doing so was the way to claim it for herself.

But perhaps the most powerful part of Yolanda's healing came in the form of someone who had died years earlier. Her great-aunt, Yolanda shared, was the only person with whom she could totally be herself. With "Tia," as she called her, she could express sorrow, as well as joy, celebrate her triumphs, and mourn her losses.

"What," I asked her, "would Tia say to you now if she were here?"

Without hesitation, Yolanda was able to recount the ways her great-aunt would love her through her pain, as she had done so many times before.

"And what would it be like if you could let yourself feel that love that you shared with Tia, and from that place, do those loving things for yourself?"

Suddenly, it was as if the lights went on for Yolanda. She realized that she had within her a way to discover who she might now become, a template to give to herself what she had, until now, only given to others. In that moment, Yolanda knew that she needed to be a loving mother to herself.

SKILL BUILDING

CHAPTER 8

1. Your "tipping point" is the time at which you know your options will need to be reassessed. If you are presently in fertility treatment, list the three considerations that you think will bring you to your tipping point. These considerations usually come under the headings of: time invested, money spent, and emotional and physical stress. Ask your husband or partner to do the same thing. Schedule time to discuss your findings together and determine how, knowing your tipping point, and your spouse's tipping point, influences each of you and how it affects your marriage. Schedule regular follow-ups together, to monitor any changes in the way either of you are feeling.

2. Yolanda's story, from the Chapter 8 case study, provides such a beautiful example of how saying good-bye is essential to moving into the next chapter of your life. Wherever you are in your fertility process, create a ritual to honor all of your dashed hopes and disappointments up until now. You can do this alone, but you may also want to consider including your husband or women friends facing similar struggles. Engage in this ritual with the intention of stepping away from what has gone before, and moving forward with renewed strength and hope.

See the

Big Picture

"More tears are shed over answered prayers than unanswered ones."

While Truman Capote had his own reasons for writing those chilling words, they do speak to an inescapable fact of life: that happiness does not necessarily occur just because everything happens the way you plan for it to happen. A broken dream that can appear devastating in the moment can sometimes turn out to have an unexpected silver lining—a gift that is not readily apparent. The truth is, a contented life happens not only when you have good days, wonderful moments, and happy events, but also when you choose to look for the opportunities, even the grace that can easily get buried under life's disappointments.

Do you remember your high school yearbook? Back in those days, it was customary, especially in senior year, for everyone to pass yearbooks around to each other so that you could write about a special time, or perhaps share a few words about how you'll remember each other. One of the common phrases you might recall was, "Don't ever change." Even though

your seventh power tool is: see the big picture

that was meant to be a compliment of sorts, think about it for a minute... you're seventeen, maybe eighteen years old, and you're telling each other never to change! Looking back on it now, this wishful thinking appears naïve, certainly shortsighted. But how many of you still believe that life can come with cruise control that lets you reach the happiness speed and then hold things there without doing anything more than occasionally guiding the steering wheel?

If you want to create a contented, rewarding life, your only option is to keep your eyes on the road; really enjoying life's straight-aways, acknowledging to yourself that there will inevitably be unexpected twists and turns. Yes, change does make for a certain amount of challenge and unpredictability. But, change can also keep life fresh and alive, and open to the possibility that there may be unexpected joy around every corner.

For some women, believing that there's a big picture beyond your longing for a pregnancy, or your dream that your family will be created in a certain way, may require a big leap of faith. You may struggle and feel compelled to ask the "why" question. The truth is, you can ask if you want to, but as Chapter 7 pointed out, this way of thinking is often circular and of little value. *Why* questions keep you in the realm of the small picture, feeling stuck and cheated. *Why* questions close the door on life's surprises, and the chance that maybe, just maybe, there's something more for you.

You have a choice. Just for today, stop asking yourself why you can't get pregnant and why this has happened to you. For one day, every time you feel the question creep into your brain, replace it with another question, an empowering one. Replace it with positive thoughts about your life, your future, or your marriage. Do this tomorrow morning, and the day after that, and every day that follows, get out of bed and try to do it again, for just one day at a time.

Your experience with infertility may be the first of life's unplanned, un-scripted challenges you face. It would be wonderful if it was the last, but if you hang around this planet long enough, that's not likely to be the case. While that may sound like a depressing thought, it does not have to be. The zingers life hands you—those things for which you have no Plan B—don't have to bring your good life to a halt.

Yes, there are life-changing events, even situations like infertility that appear devastating, and are almost-unbearably painful. The key word is "almost". You may not be able to choose whether you conceive a biologi-cal child. Your vision of yourself as a mother may very well turn out to be different from what you had planned. Nevertheless, in the big picture, you can choose whether you will forever be a victim of a situation that did not match your small picture, or whether you will be victorious in the quest to build the big picture of the good life you desire.

Redefining Fair and Unfair; Success and Failure

Conceiving a biological child may be your definition of what it would mean for your life to be successful and fair, and there is value in that. The birth of a child brings enormous blessings and you can, for a time, wrap yourself in that sweet baby smell and the wonder of someone who makes you the center of his or her world.

Again, look at the big picture. If you think about parenthood honestly, you must also acknowledge there are risks, whether they are in pregnancy, or in determining the mental and physical wellbeing of your child. There are financial risks when you think about the astronomical expense of chil-drearing. Certainly there are risks when your child gets older, becomes

every decision has gains and losses, and a small picture victory in no way translates into a big picture gain

an adolescent, and is exposed to influences well beyond your control. There are even risks relative to the success of your marriage, and whether your child will be raised in an intact home. Even if you beat all these odds and have a healthy, successful child in a happy home, a baby still means the end to that honeymoon-type freedom that childfree couples have the chance to enjoy in marriage. With the top three conflicts between married couples being sex, money, and the children, a child can become a new topic for argument with your spouse as you face the realities of rearing a child in a very challenging world.

Are any of these reasons to *not* conceive a baby if you want one? No, but they are still realities; they are still truths of life, they still happen every day. Facing these truths also can remind you that every decision has gains and losses, and that a small picture victory in no way translates into big picture success.

Giving birth to a biological child is not *succeeding* in life; it does not translate to, "happily ever after." A baby in your life is simply the accomplishment of a small picture goal, and this will inevitably pave the way to big picture issues and challenges. Admitting the realities of the big picture will require you to be brutally honest with yourself. You will be using your truth tool to its fullest extent.

But this honesty about life's fairness and unfairness will give you enormous freedom, too. You can now redefine what it means to be successful by your ability to turn challenges into opportunities for growth. The crisis of infertility can, if you let it, make you more resilient and strong. Walking through this challenge hand in hand with your partner can make your marriage better, more adaptable, and more emotionally intimate. Dealing with fertility issues can give you coping and relationship skills that you use and rely on for the rest of your life. If you let these things happen, then you will be creating your own life story of success.

As you read in the beginning of the book, the authors, Marina Lombardo and Linda J. Parker, have each faced their own life challenges. Their stories are different from yours, but in many ways, they are very much the same. They depict what is true for everyone: that the willingness to ride through life's unexpected twists and turns, and to grow from unexpected challenges, is the real measure of life's success.

Linda's Very Personal Story

I have sometimes wondered if certain events in my life were set in motion the year I was in the third grade. For many children, the third grade seems to be a transitional year, and I was no exception. It was the year I enrolled in a new school and the year I began wearing thick, heavy, bifocal glasses. I probably could not have been more intimidated by life in general.

The third grade was also the year I first encountered Mrs. Cox's class. In the small school system I attended, long before the days of special classes for every different type of special need, there was one, catch-all class for students with handicaps and disabilities. The class was known simply as, "Mrs. Cox's retarded class" and for one entire year, I watched them from afar, frightened and disturbed by the students I saw.

Today, I look back in amazement that one teacher could handle a class-room of both elementary and secondary school students whose disabilities ranged from mild to severe. In hindsight, I believe she not only managed the class with a great deal of love, but she did it extraordinarily well. Yet at the time, I was oblivious to the positive things that were going on in her classroom; I was simply alarmed and confused by these children (many of whom were nearing adulthood) who spoke, walked, talked, and ate in ways that were different from anyone I had seen before. And ironically, it was the way they ate that created the most distress for me.

Our school cafeteria was a basement room, and not particularly conducive to pleasant lunches even under the best of circumstances. Because my class was on schedule to eat each day at the same time Mrs. Cox's class ate, the two classes usually occupied two long rows of tables facing one another.

If you were a third grader near the front of the daily lunch line, you could grab a seat facing your own classmates, not the students in Mrs. Cox's class. Unfortunately, I was never near the front of the lunch line. In order to claim such a coveted spot, you had to be willing to push ahead of the other children at the exact moment you turned the corner and were—for a few brief seconds—out of your teacher's sight.

I could never do that. I was a rule-follower and could not bring myself to disobey my teacher's warnings about running inside the school. Besides, there was always the matter of my knee socks.

My legs were skinny and there was absolutely no way knee socks were going to stay anywhere near my knees. Instead, my socks "puddled" around my bony ankles, leaving my scraped, bruised, and comically thin legs exposed to weather and ridicule. (Scraped and bruised must be a universal description of the knees and elbows of children who view life through bifocal glasses). As I walked through the corridors of my elementary school, the process involved taking approximately two steps forward and then bending over to pull up my socks. Two more steps and it was time to pull up my socks again. There wasn't a chance I was ever going to make it to the front of any line.

For nine painfully long months spent in the third grade, I ate my lunch every day, facing the students in Mrs. Cox's class. I watched with a child's honest

acceptance gives us the permission we need to start loving our imperfect life just because it is our life, and ours alone

repulsion as Mrs. Cox's students drooled and slobbered their way through their meals. I don't think I swallowed a bite during that entire school year, no doubt, making my legs even skinnier.

But third grade eventually turned into fourth, and my lunch schedule was no longer in sync with that of Mrs. Cox. In time, I went off to junior high school, traded knee socks for pantyhose, and the freedom to wear slacks to school. Life in general got a whole lot better.

Years later, in college, I studied fine arts and earned a certificate to teach both high school and elementary school students. I took special classes in order to work with hearing impaired students, and night classes to certify me to teach adults. I covered all the bases of people I might teach, except for mentally retarded students—or as they had been relabeled by that time, special needs students. I did not want to be around those children who looked and acted so differently from the rest of us.

So how do I get from that place in my life, to telling you that I am blessed to be the mother of a special needs—no, a mentally retarded child? Not easily, I assure you. But I will start by mentioning that life does not always turn out like you expect.

My beautiful daughter was born several weeks prematurely. She was tiny and thin, and cried louder than any other baby in the nursery. My doctors said she would be fine. Her delivery was quick and relatively un-complicated, although it was a breeched birth, a fact that my obstetrician failed to realize until the final minutes before my daughter entered this world. Fortunately, her lungs were fully developed; she could breathe on her own, and she was ready to eat the moment she arrived. Seven days after her birth, I took my four pound, nine ounce baby home.

I've never known if my daughter earned her good APGAR results,[10] or if they were "awarded" as a way to diminish the chances of me, years later, filing a medical malpractice lawsuit related to her delivery. I won't go into the details to rehash the years of her life that were spent in the offices of doctors, psychologists, and therapists of every sort. Nor will I enumerate the number of times my child's brain was scanned, viewed, photographed, analyzed, or tested.

I have often thought that being her mother would have been easier if, on day-1 in the hospital, someone had said to me, "Your child was born with X-Y-Z disease." But no one did that. For seventeen years of her life, no one could tell me what was wrong or why there were problems. No authority I looked to could tell me what my daughter might be able to do as she matured and what would be outside her capabilities. By this time, I was a single mother (also not part of my life plan) with two beautiful little girls born fifteen months apart, one of whom had an un-diagnosable condition. Not the limbo of infertility, but certainly a gray area of unknowing, that in my case lasted seventeen years.

My little daughters and I flew without a net. We charted unknown waters every day and I spent more time fighting with school administrators than you can imagine. In some ways, life was about as difficult as it could possibly be, until it got worse.

In the years between thirty-something and forty-something, I was diagnosed not once, but twice with life-threatening illnesses and given dismal to no odds of surviving. But I didn't have time to be sick. I was the mother,

---

[10] APGAR is the evaluation used at birth to assess the overall health of a newborn.

father, caregiver, and breadwinner all rolled into one. I was my daughter's advocate. I carried the responsibility of making sure that my "unlabeled" child got every opportunity she could and that no one presumed her limitations and created any more stumbling blocks for her than she already faced. I also carried the responsibility to make life as normal as possible for her bright, precocious little sister, who did not deserve to grow up in the shadow of her sister's handicap. Very little about my life was going according to plan.

My first breakthrough happened in December of 1980, when my daughter was nine months old. I certainly did not feel like celebrating the upcoming holidays. I had a child who cried too much, slept too little, and was not hitting her developmental milestones on schedule. I had some of the best doctors in the country giving me "non-answers" as to why. And I was pregnant again, in a marriage I was already sure was a mistake. I had no idea if my second child would face the challenges my first child was dealing with, because no one knew what had gone wrong the first time. But Christmas was coming whether I wanted it to or not and some preparations were inevitable. So I bundled my tiny little daughter in pink fleece baby bunting and went out into the world to shop.

To my eyes, every store in the mall might as well have had a big sign that read, "Christmas toys for normal children." Every child I saw waiting in line to talk to Santa looked bright, healthy, and as far as I was concerned, had a genius I.Q. After an hour or so, I'd had all I could stand. I found the elevator in a large department store and headed for the ladies room on the second floor. Forget about using the bathroom; I was just going upstairs to cry.

In the privacy of the handicapped stall, large enough for me to roll the baby stroller in with me, I took a few minutes and let tears of frustration—

at this point, for the millionth time, run down my face. Then I powdered my nose, hugged my wide-eyed baby, and tried to compose myself to finish my shopping. However, what I heard only made it more difficult.

A mother and her young daughter were chatting together as they entered the restroom. I could not see them, but their words and happy tones told me all I thought I needed to know. Here was one more mother who had gotten what women want, expect, and feel is their entitlement—a pregnancy that results in a normal, healthy child.

As much as I resented their happy exchange, I couldn't stay in the handicapped stall forever. I pushed the stroller toward the row of sinks. The perfect mother and perfect daughter were washing their hands as I approached. The little girl stood with her back to me, but I could see her wool coat and matching hat, both red with black velvet trim, and I could hear her talking enthusiastically about the cookies they were going to bake.

I waited to take my place at the sink, waited for them to go away and get out of my sight, and waited for the resentment I felt to subside, even though I knew it wouldn't. But as the woman and her daughter turned to leave, I saw the little girl's face for the first time. Beautiful curls framed her pink cheeks, and she smiled at me broadly. I could only stare back at her, dumbfounded, with my mouth wide open.

The "perfect" little girl had Down syndrome.

I will never know if her mother had divine insight to understand my rudeness, or if, in her years of mothering this child, she had simply developed her own way to cope. Yet, as I stood there, confused by my own incorrect assumptions, saying nothing at all, the woman looked at me and said, "God picks special mothers to have special children."

In that awkward moment, this stranger gave me the words I needed to hear. She gave me an answer that filled the questioning void in my mind in a way that nothing else had been able to do. Of course, her statement doesn't bear itself out under the scrutiny of pure logic. Obviously all children are special and it is equally obvious that special needs children are unfortunately born to neglectful mothers all the time. Likewise, women who would be fantastic mothers to a disabled or handicapped child may have totally healthy children or may have no children at all. Nevertheless, the comfort, I gained from her statement was the simple message that we don't have to know the plan, or even understand it. Just to accept that there is a plan, even when it doesn't make sense to us, and even when it is not the plan we wanted for ourselves. The little girl's mother wasn't speaking to the logical part of me; she was speaking to my heart. In that moment, I immediately understood that I could make my life miserable or I could accept the situation and then strive to actually become my special daughter's special mother. The operative word is "accept".

With acceptance comes remarkable healing. Acceptance brings the freedom to step out of the quagmire and move forward. Acceptance gives us the permission we need to start loving our imperfect life just because it is our life and ours alone. Perfection within our life is not what makes it meaningful and special. Our lives are—with all their flaws—extraordinary because they are our own personal canvas on which to paint, write, and create. We are never too young, too old, too broken, too failed, or too alone to reinvent ourselves. Painting the picture we envisioned is far less important than finding joy in the act of putting paint on the canvas.

I mentioned that my daughter was seventeen years old before I first got answers, and even then, the answers were vague. I will always remember the day my daughters were curling their hair and putting on mascara to have graduation pictures taken. Each was starting her last year in high school. My younger daughter was a senior at the local public school and my older daughter was a senior at the special school she attended. And it happened in a flash.

My older daughter slumped to floor, twitching slightly all over. It was her first seizure and it drove the two of us back to more doctors and more tests. Technology had improved since her most recent CAT scans and MRI's, some five years earlier. From the test results, I learned that some damage had occurred during my daughter's birth and also that her brain was malformed. My beautiful daughter, who I love with all my heart, was not merely slow or challenged. She was mentally retarded, just like the students in Mrs. Cox's class.

I had inhaled seventeen years earlier and only with that news began to exhale. The words I had tried so hard to avoid became my ultimate reality. All of the years that I had breathed a sigh of relief because brain damage and retardation were not our diagnosis were wiped out in a single moment sitting in the doctor's office. I not only had to face the leviathan that had lurked in my path for so long, I had to step into all of my raw-edged emotions and accept both my reality and my daughter's.

So what happened next?

The second step of my "breakthrough". Slowly, I began to tell people in my life about my daughter. When I met new acquaintances, I learned to say, "I have two daughters, one is in college and the other is mentally handicapped and is at home with me."

I found that putting it out there and making it a little more upfront in my life, not only helped me come to terms with the diagnosis, but also circumvented the awkwardness that inevitably occurred later because someone felt bad for saying the wrong thing at the wrong time. I was learning to tell myself and others the authentic truth.

I also learned that there are no perfect families. Every single person has challenges—usually tough ones—to face in life. People have children they don't want and people want children they can't have. Healthy children die young and brilliant children make disastrous choices in life. The point is, none of us ever has that perfect life we dream we will have. We have a life, filled with disappointments, imperfections, and a limitless potential for personal happiness. The choice of which part of it we choose to focus our energy and our attention, is a choice no one else can make for us. We can step up to the challenge to live a rich full life or we can choose to let events outside of our control dictate the quality of our days.

And then what happened after that?

After what felt like a hundred years of being single, I met and married a man who loves me and all my imperfections—a man I love so much he takes my breath away every time he walks into the room.

So has my life been a case of, "what we resist persists?" In some ways, "yes". And I am the first to tell you that my life hasn't turned out at all as I imagined it would when I was sixteen or twenty-one, or even thirty-nine.

Parts of my life have been challenging and very painful. And other parts of my life have been more richly blessed and profoundly happy than I ever thought was possible. After all these years, I still have days when I grieve the loss of the person my daughter might have been, or I am overwhelmed by concerns about who will be her caregiver as I grow older and what will be the quality of her life if I am not around. While the greater part of my grief has passed, I accept the fact that some aspects of grief never leave you. I'm okay with that and when I feel the sadness, I treat myself gently.

I also have feelings of self-pity at times because I just want to go out for dinner alone with my husband or get away for the weekend and arranging who will take care of my daughter is sometimes so difficult that it becomes easy to abandon my social plans. When this happens, I try not to run from these feelings; that only gives them reason to chase me. Instead, I turn and face them. I allow my emotional experiences to guide me.

Inevitably, as my feelings come into perspective, my issues begin to seem very manageable. Having survived a lot gives you an amazing kind of confidence. Over the years, I have learned the ingredients for my own personal prescription for peace. It usually includes small pleasures like incredible French soap or books by favorite authors who take me outside myself. Often it involves making a deliberate effort to help someone else; giving to others is one of the greatest self-help strategies available. Always it involves prayer.

Serenity happens when I make conscious choices that are truly right for me. The secret is that it is most likely to happen when I can step outside myself and realize that life isn't really all about me. When I do that, I can perceive my experiences, not as crises, but as the opportunities for personal growth that they have proven to be.

Marina's Very Personal Story

In the beginning of this book, I shared with you that striving for a child is an issue that is very close to my heart. I personally know the feeling of wanting a child so much, that I was willing to do almost anything to make it happen.

As the mother of both an adopted child and a biological child, my dream turned out a little differently than what I had originally planned. But within that challenge came an unexpected gift. What I discovered was that, for me, there was no difference between adoption and biology. When they handed me my son, and later, my daughter, my heart was filled with that same indescribable mother's love each time.

You see, I was never the kind of young person who was instinctively drawn to children. I never did much babysitting,

gratitude is humility in action

and the few times I was left with a baby or toddlers, I found myself both exhausted and exasperated, counting the minutes to their bedtime. As an insecure teenager, I was often annoyed by what others considered to be their irresistible cuteness, and since I saw them as competition for attention, my strategy was to do my best to ignore them. I share all this to illustrate just how out of character it was for me, while in the midst of this time of my life, to decide that one day not only would I adopt a child, but also get a glimpse of what my future family would look like.

It was 1972, and I was just nineteen years old. Anyone who has been on Long Island in early summer can tell you that this is the time of year when days are tailored to perfection—clear skies that go on forever, no humidity at all. On such a day, my friend Susan asked if I wanted to spend the weekend with her older brother, who lived with his family in upstate New York. Sure, nothing else was going on. Susan was quite a bit older than I, an old hippie really, and our pairing was a bit unusual. Still, we always had an easy friendship, and the ride up was no exception. I spotted the two boys first, roughhousing in the driveway, playing basketball. Handsome boys, clean, all American looking, both around middle school age. Good kids too, as I recall—well mannered, and versed in making small talk with adults. When I met their parents, it was easy to see where they had gotten their good looks, and their easy manner.

I spent some time getting acclimated and settled in my room before being introduced to the family's youngest member, a little girl, no more than two years old. I can still remember my reaction when I first saw her. Speechless, I felt like I was looking at an angel. Her dark hair and eyes, her olive skin, in contrast to her brothers, told of her adoption. Petite, delicate, she had a sense of self-awareness, a presence about her that I had never noticed in a child—but then again, I had barely noticed children at all! Later that evening, when we all gathered in the living room after dinner, I found it difficult to look away from her. I watched her laugh when her father tickled her, her look of consternation when her brother teased, how she examined a toy before deciding whether to play with it or not. I was totally and completely smitten, and no one was more surprised than I was. This, I decided, is what my family would look like someday—a blend of biological and adopted children.

Years passed, and eventually I met my future husband. As we got to know one another, I shared with him my vision for my family, and he was on board, wholeheartedly. Wonderful, I recall thinking—a partner who can share the same dream. As I look back on it now, however, I realize how little I knew. Yes, my dream would eventually come to fruition, but the road there would look different from anything I could imagine.

We were married three years when I became pregnant with my son. For the first few months, the pregnancy went smoothly. I can still see myself waiting for the OB to come into the examining room thinking smugly to myself, "I am such a boring patient!" And thankfully, as far as the pregnancy went, I was.

But there came a day, sometime during my mid second trimester, when the ease of my pregnancy became a thing of the past. I was at work, standing in a long hallway, preparing to deliver a message to a colleague, when I turned and suddenly felt a shift in my lower back, a pain that screamed down the right side of my body. I stood frozen for a minute, afraid to move. When I finally caught my breath, the pain didn't leave, and in fact, seared down my leg with every step I took.

To say that this came out of nowhere wouldn't be exactly right. I had always had a sensitive back, a structural issue that was congenital. When I was a child, I would strain my back doing things that other kids would find easy—vacuuming floors, or leaning over a bit too long. But it never caused a real problem, and usually, I'd be able to just shake it out, and it would adjust itself. This time, however, there was no "shaking it out." When I told my OB about it hoping for an answer, he simply shrugged, and chalked it up to "a bit of sciatica" as a result of the pregnancy. That was no consolation, and a haze of pain clouded the rest of my pregnancy. Oftentimes, it was hard for me to stand erect, and I realize I must have been quite a sight, pregnant as I was, hunched over, and limping.

Finally, my beautiful son Michael was born. But the joy that should have sustained me was compromised by unrelenting pain. Don't get me wrong—some days were better than others were for sure. In my mind, though, I had an image of returning to how I felt even before I became pregnant, and felt frustrated that so much of my caregiving had to be managed around my physical limitations.

When my son was just a few months old, I decided to start seeking real answers for my pain. Neurologists, orthopedists, chiropractors, massage therapists; I tried them all, carting my baby from appointment to appointment. After about a year of virtually no relief, a neurosurgeon recommended a surgery to alleviate the pressure he felt the spinal discs were putting on my nerves, as well as to shorten a bone he thought might be creating an imbalance in my back. I knew this was a big step, but I was desperate and willing to try anything. What I did not realize were the risks involved.

Arriving at the hospital early on the morning before my surgery, I should have paid attention to my first clue. There was empty space where a bed should have been, and as I waited for the bed's delivery from another place in the hospital, a small voice inside my head kept saying, "It's a sign. You shouldn't be here. Get out!" A feeling of dread fell over me. I took a deep breath and tried to shake it off. Just nerves, I told myself. The next morning, the surgery went off as scheduled.

My hospital bed was pushed up against a glass wall, looking out on to the nurse's station. I can still see myself lying there, waking up after the surgery, groggy and hooked up to an IV of pain medication. Strangely, I was unable to move. For the next five days, I lay there, floating in and out of consciousness, practically immobile. Although I found it hard to hold on to a coherent thought, there was one thing I do remember thinking— something was wrong. When I was finally able to get out of bed, my body felt so painful, so rigid, it was as though it belonged to someone else. By the time I left the hospital ten days later, every movement was an effort. I had to learn to walk all over again.

I've always been a great believer that when one door closes, another opens, and my stay at the hospital was no exception. Remember, I still had my son at home, and one of my worries was how I would be able to care for him. My husband was doing his best to rearrange his schedule, but there would be times that he just couldn't be there. As synchronicity would have it, my hospital roommate was a lovely young woman, there for a minor hernia surgery. As we became acquainted, she shared that she would be out of work for a while to recover. Would she be interested in coming over a few hours every day and helping with my son? He was almost two years old, and even though he was pretty adept at getting himself in and out of things, he needed someone who could look after him. Thankfully, she said yes.

Recovery was slow, painstakingly slow. The doctors didn't have much to say. Something about, "We had to do more than we anticipated," and "These types of things have risks," and of course, my favorite, "Well, of course, now there's scar tissue to deal with." At one point, about a year after the surgery, I decided to see a top neurosurgeon in New York City for a second opinion, bringing my pre and post surgical cat scans. All he could do was shake his head.

But at thirty-one years old, I still had a lot of life ahead of me, and I was determined not to live with disability. Yes, often I felt bitter and frustrated. And like anyone else, I often sang the familiar refrain, "Why me?" But I knew there was only so far that line of thinking would take me, and I was determined not to make this way of being my home. I started by swimming, literally counting strokes until I could swim a lap. I started walking, first to the end of the driveway, then to the corner of the street, until I reached a mile. I started practicing yoga, Pilates; anything that I thought would help strengthen my back. I sought the treatment of a wonderful cranial osteopath who helped me to regain some mobility in my spine. No, I wasn't what I was—and over the years, I was able to accept that I would never be that person again. But I was healthy; I was stronger, and one step at a time, I was getting my life back.

Around this time, my husband and I started talking about another child. Another pregnancy was unadvisable, the doctors said—there was no telling how my back would respond. So, we decided we would do what we had planned from the start—we would adopt. A year later, our beautiful daughter Melissa became part of our family. That was over twenty years ago, but even as I write this now, I get tears in my eyes. Because, you see, dreams do come true, even though how we get there may look so different than we ever imagined.

Often, I've asked myself what I've gained as a result of the road I've traveled. Well, I know I have tremendous respect for the resilience of my physical wellbeing. I know I have so much more sensitivity and compassion for anyone who struggles with disability, limitation, with a body that seems to have a mind of its own. I realize that, even though I didn't know it at the time, the experience has given me the heart and passion for the clinical work I do today, especially with fertility clients. I know I have grown spiritually, and I now see how life can transform a self-centered young woman, into a mother for whom adoption or biology made no difference at all.

And I got to have my family—the family I always wanted. The morning we picked up Melissa is as clear now as the day it happened. She was just a few weeks old when I met her, and from the first moment I saw her, I was speechless, as though I was looking at an angel. She was petite, delicate, with dark hair, olive skin, and a presence about her that I had never noticed in a child—not since that fateful day many years before.

Trying times, desperate times—everyone has them, and there are moments when every single one of us is tempted just to give up. Sometimes it is all you can do simply to put one step in front of the other—and sometimes doing simply this is enough. But to make this choice a lifestyle is a loss—for you and all that you could be.

You are not alone on your journey. The tools presented in this book are here to support you, to guide you, and to help you turn any challenge into an opportunity for growth. As I look back on my own story, I see the price I paid for the times I ignored their wisdom, as well as the benefits I gained when I followed through. For example, I remember how I pushed myself to keep going during my pregnancy, as if giving into my pain would have been an acknowledgement, even a defeat of sorts. How I wish now that I had slowed down and listened to my body, and given it the care it so desperately needed. I recall the ambivalence I had about having the surgery, knowing even through my desperation, that this choice was not right for me. And yet, I did not listen to my own truth, and even the morning of arrival at the hospital, turned away from making a conscious choice that I knew was right for me. Powerful lessons that taught me the dire consequences of turning away from myself, and how important it was to do what was right for me. But within the pain of these losses, I also learned the lessons of grief. By honoring grief and embracing it, I finally was able to see the big picture. I could clearly envision the steps to creating a new, rich, and rewarding life.

If you are grieving the loss of the family you had hoped for, or if you are in the midst of fertility treatment, uncertain how to move forward—take heart. Know that within the very challenge you are facing are the seeds to a new life that is waiting for you. See the big picture and know that this life may not look, or feel like anything you had ever imagined—but it may well be greater than anything for which you could have ever hoped.

The Really Big Picture

Sometimes, when you are in the middle of a tough situation, it's easy to forget what life was like before, and imagine that your struggle will go on forever. But the most hopeful thing to understand is that this time in your life will end—it is, by its very nature, time-limited. If you are committed to having a family, you will have one. It may not look the way you think it will today, but it could very well turn out to be more than anything you can imagine.

The big picture—the really big picture—says that the very challenge you are struggling with right now brings with it gifts and opportunities. These

know that within the very challenge you are facing are the seeds of a new life waiting for you opportunities are present in your life *because* of what you are experiencing. Ask to be able to see them, to recognize them for the gifts they are. Ask to be shown how to grow into them, to use them to become more than what you thought you could be.

Prolific American author and intellectual, Joseph Campbell made an observation that probably says it best. His words are wisdom to live by, now and for the rest of your life: "We must be willing to let go of the life we have planned so as to have the life that is waiting for us."

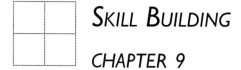

SKILL BUILDING

CHAPTER 9

1. Moving outside yourself is powerful. The moment you stop living your life
    focused only on your own situation, and focus on someone else, you gain
    incredible freedom from the weight that is bearing down so heavily on your
    shoulders. This is because of the connection we all share with one another.
    In extending love or simply compassion to someone else, even in the
    simplest of ways, you are in fact, reaping the rewards of that which you give.

Right now, make a list of small ways you can step outside yourself, take the
magnifying glass off your struggle, and reach out to someone else. Can you
telephone someone you know who is lonely and will appreciate your call? When
you pick up a mug of gourmet coffee tomorrow morning, can you also get one
for the new assistant at your workplace? Can you remember to hold the door
for someone the next time you go shopping, or give a warm smile to the person
next to you at the checkout line?

2. Choose one item from your list and commit to implementing it today.
    Expand your list, and commit to doing one thing each day—no matter how
    insignificant you believe it is. There is truly a cumulative value to giving, and a
    momentum that builds when you live with an open heart.

3. Keep your journal by your bed, and each night, note not only the ways
    in which you have given, but also list what two or three things you have
    received or for which you have to be grateful. They can be things that
    specifically happened that day, or general things that are easy to overlook
    and take for granted.

There is an Attitudinal Healing Principle that says, "Giving and receiving are
the same." As you pick up this thread by reaching out to others, you not only
enlarge your world, you open the doors of the universe to receive.

Are You Interested in More?

*More growth…more self-understanding…*and more ways to take turn the life crisis of infertility into a personal breakthrough?

I Am More Than My Infertility Personal Breakthrough Tool Kit will help you take Marina Lombardo's 7 proven tools to a deeper, more personal level of use.

Your toolkit is a 7-step plan, packed with worksheets, audio files, slides, personal assessments, and charts, all especially designed to support you and your emotional needs as you face the challenges of infertility. The Tool Kit is your companion as you begin, from wherever you are, to move toward peace and clarity, and create the fulfilling, satisfying life you deserve.

Visit either of the following websites to order your tool kit now, or to learn more about how ***I Am More Than My Infertility Personal Breakthrough Tool Kit*** can help you transform your life challenges into a time of incredible personal growth and meaning:

www.IAmMore.net

www.MarinaLombardo.com

BIBLIOGRAPHY

Benson, Herbert, M. *Beyond the Relaxation Response.* New York: Times Books, 1984.

Benson, Herbert, M. *The Relaxation Response.* New York: Harper Collins, 1975.

Brizendine, Louann, MD. *The Female Brain.* New York: Broadway, (Random House) 2006.

Carter, Jean and Michael. Sweet Grapes, *How to Stop Being Infertile and Start Living Again.* Indiana: Perspectives Press, Expanded edition, 1998.

Domar, Alice D., and Kelly, Alice Lesch. *Conquering Infertility: Dr. Alice Domar's Mind/Body Guide to Enhancing Fertility and Coping with Infertility.* New York: Penguin Group, 2002.

Geary, Amanda. *The Mind Guide to Food and Mood.* (Booklet) London: Mind, 2000, 2004.

Geary, Amanda. *The Food and Mood Handbook.* UK: Thorsons (HarperCollins), 2001.

Gendlin, Eugene, PhD. *Focusing.* New York: Bantam revised edition, May 1981.

Greenberg, Leslie S., PhD. *Emotion-Focused Therapy: Coaching Clients to Work Through Their Feelings.* Washington, D.C: American Psychological Association, 2002.

Hendricks, Gay. *The Ten Second Miracle: Creating Relationship Breakthroughs.* New York: Harper Collins, 1998.

Hendricks, Gay and Hendricks, Kathlyn, Ph.D. *At The Speed of Life.* New York: Bantam Books, 1993.

Hendricks, Gay and Kathlyn, Ph.D. *Conscious Loving, The Journey to Co-Commitment.* New York: Bantam Books, 1992.

Hogan, Kevin. *The Psychology of Persuasion.* Louisiana: Pelican Publishing, 1996.

Katherine, Ann, M.A. *Boundaries, Where You End and I Begin.* New York: Simon and Schuster, Fireside Books, 1991. (Fireside Reissue, 2000).

Parker, Linda J. *The San of Africa.* Minnesota: Lerner Publications. Singapore: Times Publishing Group, 2002.

Payne, Niravi B. M.S. and Richardson, Brenda Lane. *The Whole Person Fertility Program* sm. New York: Three Rivers Press, 1997.

Progoff, Ira. *At a Journal Workshop.* New York: Dialogue House Library, 1975.

Progoff, Ira. *The Practice of Process Meditation.* New York: Dialogue House Library, 1980.

Rainer, Maria Rilke. *Letters to a Young Poet.* California: New World Library, 2002.

Seftel, Laura. *Grief Unseen: Healing Pregnancy Loss Through The Arts.* Philadelphia, Pennsylvania: Jessica Kingsley Publishers, 2006.

Thoele, Sue Patton. *The Woman's Book of Spirit: Meditations for the Thirsty Soul.* California: Conari Press, 2006.

Willard, Terry, Ph.D. *Mind-Body Harmony How to Resist and Recover from Auto-Immune Diseases,* Toronto: Sarasota Press, 2002.

RECOMMENDED RESOURCES

I AM MORE

http://www.IAmMore.net

A website for women, by women, and about women, created to provide support, education, community, and a safe place to land, in today's hectic and demanding world. At the **I Am More** website, you can sign up to receive Marina Lombardo's newsletter, *Seeds of Growth*. You can participate in ongoing research surveys about women's experiences with fertility challenges; listen to Marina's internet radio broadcasts, and read "Emotionally Speaking," Marina's column that appears in *Conceive* magazine.

You can order *I Am More Than My Infertility: 7 Proven Tools for Turning a Life Crisis into a Personal Breakthrough*, and the *I Am More Than My Infertility Personal Breakthrough Tool Kit* at **www.IAmMore.net** or **www.MarinaLombardo.com**. Available as a downloadable learning program, the *I Am More Than My Infertility Personal Breakthrough Tool Kit*, helps you take Marina Lombardo's 7 proven tools to a deeper, more personal level of use as you turn the life crisis of infertility into your own breakthrough.

Your toolkit is a 7-step plan designed with you in mind, to support your emotional needs as you face the challenges of infertility. The Tool Kit includes worksheets, audio files, slides, personal assessments, and charts. The Tool Kit is your companion as you begin, from wherever you are, to move toward peace and clarity, and create the fulfilling, satisfying life you deserve.

Marina Lombardo

http://www.MarinaLombardo.com

The professional website for Marina Lombardo, LCSW, PA, where you can learn more about Marina—her credentials and private clinical and personal coaching practice. You can also access the archive of Marina's *Seeds of Growth* newsletters, her "Emotionally Speaking" columns that have appeared in *Conceive Magazine*, and her internet radio broadcasts that have aired on *Conceive on Air.*

Most importantly, you can learn more about Marina's personal and professional philosophy: that the very challenges you are facing in life are not obstacles, but invitations to step into a larger sense of yourself—that they are, in fact, opportunities for growth.

Conceive Magazine

http://www.conceiveonline.com

Conceive Magazine is the first and only publication created for women as a fertility lifestyle magazine. *Conceive Magazine,* and the companion website *ConceiveOnline,* offer information and support for women and their partners on the journey to creating families.

Also visit *Conceive On Air* at:

http://www.modavox.com/modaview/conceiveonair/

INCIID

The InterNational Council on Infertility Information Dissemination

http://www.inciid.org/

INCIID (pronounced "Inside") is a nonprofit organization that provides links to the latest, medically responsible information on the Internet for people experiencing infertility.

RESOLVE

The National Infertility Association

http://www.resolve.org

RESOLVE is a non-profit organization that offers nationwide chapters to provide support and information to people dealing with infertility, as well as increase public awareness of infertility issues through advocacy and public education.

ASRM

American Society of Reproductive Medicine

http://www.asrm.org

ASRM is a professional organization committed to advancing information and expertise in reproductive medicine by serving as an advocate for patient care, research, and education, and developing education materials for professionals and patients.

ADOPTIVE FAMILIES MAGAZINE

http:///www.adoptivefamilies.com

An award-winning national magazine, *Adoptive Families* provides information for families before, during and after adoption, as well as an annual guide featuring the most current how-to-adopt information.

BIOGRAPHY OF DR. MARK P. TROLICE

Mark P. Trolice, M.D., FACOG, FACS, FACE is the Director of Fertility C.A.R.E. (Center of Assisted Reproduction & Endocrinology) as well as the Division Director of Reproductive Endocrinology & Infertility (REI), at Orlando Regional Healthcare in Florida, responsible for the medical education of Obstetrics and Gynecology (OB/GYN) resident physicians and third/fourth year medical students in REI. Additionally, Dr. Trolice is a Clinical Associate Professor in the Department of OB/GYN at the University of Florida in Gainesville and Florida State University.

Dr. Trolice is double Board-certified in REI and OB/GYN and maintains annual voluntary recertification in these specialties and has been awarded the American Medical Association's "Physicians' Recognition Award" annually. In May 2005, Dr. Trolice was inducted into the prestigious American College of Endocrinology adding to his unique distinction of also being a fellow in the American College of OB/GYN and the American College of Surgeons.

Dr. Trolice has authored research studies and published in several leading medical journals and a textbook. He has lectured at numerous physician conferences and patient seminars around the country. In addition to participating on TV news/talk shows, radio, the internet and in the newspaper for 'expert' interviews on reproductive health topics, Dr. Trolice is on the Medical Advisory Board of *Conceive Magazine* and Central Florida Doctor Magazine. In 2004, he founded Fertile Dreams, Inc. a non-for-profit organization dedicated to increasing fertility awareness and granting scholarship for those unable to afford fertility treatment by sponsoring an annual Fertility Awareness Health Fair and Embracing Hope Gala in Orlando, FL.

Printed in the United States
152768LV00002B/11/A

9 780980 026603